PREGNANCY

AND LIFE-STYLE HABITS

PREGNANCY

AND LIFE-STYLE HABITS

PETER A. FRIED PhD

BEAUFORT BOOKS
New York • Toronto

Library of Congress Cataloging in Publication Data

Fried, Peter.
Pregnancy and life-style habits.

Bibliography: p.
Includes index.
1. Fetus—Effects of drugs on.   2. Pregnant women—Drug use.
I. Title.
RG627.6.D79F74   1983   618.3'2   83-2650
ISBN 0-8253-0151-3

Published in the United States by Beaufort Books,
New York. Published simultaneously in Canada by
General Publishing Co. Limited

Printed in Canada   First Edition
10 9 8 7 6 5 4 3 2 1

Contents

Preface

I have heard it said that writing a book is much like giving birth. Given my genetic fate, I will never be an authority on this analogy, but from the male point of view, the comparison appears appropriate. And the topic of this book makes it tempting to pursue the analogy.

First comes conception. The germ of the idea had been lying in the back of my mind for a long time. The impetus for putting pen to paper came from a number of mothers-to-be involved in a large-scale study, being conducted under my direction in Ottawa, that is investigating some of the effects of soft drugs, such as nicotine, alcohol, and caffeine when taken during pregnancy. Most of these women have questions about these widely used, self-administered drugs, and many have mentioned the difficulty of finding in-depth information written in non-technical language.

After conception comes the period of the carrying and nurturing of the developing "baby." During this period of planning, researching, and writing, the author experiences huge fluctuations of emotions: satisfaction, discouragement, highs, lows, anticipation, doubts, and fulfillment. There is no turning back. Once started, you can no more leave a chapter half-completed than you can remain half-pregnant.

As the product gets bigger and bigger, concern about the outcome grows. Will it be everything one hopes? Should something else be done or not done in order to improve it?

. If this book succeeds in answering your questions, in giving you new information about an issue that concerns you, in bridging the gap between the researcher and you, then it has accomplished the purpose it was conceived for.

The analogy between this book and a child breaks down in one important area. The responsibility for a pregnancy is obviously a shared one. *Pregnancy and Life-Style Habits* is different. Only I am responsible for the views expressed, the interpretation of the data, and any errors in fact.

Having said that, I must, however, also acknowledge the debt I owe to a large number of people. Some I do not know personally. This group includes many of the scientists whose reports in the professional literature form the basis of much of this book. Other parts of it reflect discussions with friends and colleagues in the department of psychology at Carleton University and the departments of obstetrics and gynecology of the Ottawa Civic Hospital and the Ottawa General Hospital. I owe a particular debt of gratitude to the members of my research team—dubbed the Baby Group—who have provided investigative expertise, unfailing support, and so many stimulating discussions over the past few years. Among them are Marg Buckingham, Elizabeth Drake, Joanne Gusella, Heather Lintell, Nancy Staisey, Barb Watkinson, and Ellen Williams. Appreciation is also extended to Marlene Hewitt and Cindy Reid for the typing and retyping of many drafts.

As for so much of my other work, I must express deep appreciation and affection to my wife, Elfie, for her patience, critical comments, and, most importantly, moral support during the preparation of this book.

Last, but certainly far from least, a very profound debt is owed to the many mothers-to-be and mothers-who-are with whom I have had the privilege of working over the past years. It is they, above all, who have provided the inspiration for the chapters that follow.

Introduction

If you are pregnant or have a close friend or relative who is pregnant, you have undoubtedly become aware of the large number of things people recommend avoiding during that nine-month period. It's a long, almost impossible list. This book is not meant to be a further recitation of forbidden fruits for mothers-to-be. The following chapters give facts, not scare messages or extreme statements based on speculation, about a class of substances that share one thing in common. They are all nonessentials for survival that have become, to varying degrees, part of almost everyone's life-style. These substances include alcohol, caffeine, nicotine, marijuana, and various medicines, many of them nonprescription. All of them are, of course, drugs.

This book makes no attempt to judge the wisdom of the pervasiveness of these drugs. It does not even try to tell the reader which aspects of her life-style should be changed once she becomes pregnant. The following chapters simply present, assess, and comment on what is known and what is not known about these substances when they are used during pregnancy. Given this material, which is derived from research laboratories and hospitals around the world, the mother-to-be can decide in a rational, informed way whether her dietary and life-style habits risk affecting her unborn baby.

THE NEED FOR THIS BOOK

As women take a more active and informed role during pregnancy, they demand answers to more and more questions about everyday life-style. But surprisingly, there is no in-depth, popular study of common nonessential drugs used during pregnancy. Several books about prenatal and baby care do contain passing references, but they are always couched in vague generalities and do not touch on many of the questions mothers-to-be most want answers to. Some of the issues have also begun to turn up in the general media—television documentaries, newspapers, and magazines. However, the dictates of time and space limit these forms of communication to items that make headlines, and even those subjects have to be so condensed that some distortion of the facts is almost inevitable.

Obviously, the individual mother-to-be ought to consult her own physician about the impact that particular drugs may have on her unborn baby. However, doctors must deal with such an enormous volume of information that it is unrealistic to expect the average general practitioner or obstetrician to have an in-depth knowledge of all aspects of all substances that patients may use or be exposed to during pregnancy. Studies conducted during the 1970s in North America and the British Isles estimate that 97 percent of women use prescribed drugs—an average of five to ten of them—during pregnancy. The number of nonprescription drugs is, of course, much larger and includes many substances that few laypeople think of as drugs. A very abbreviated list of the categories of drugs ingested during pregnancy includes iron and vitamin supplements, appetite suppressants, over-the-counter painkillers and cough medicines, barbiturates, hormones, tranquilizers, antacids, antibiotics, and the drugs of social use—nicotine, alcohol, caffeine, and marijuana.

Information about the effects of these and other substances comes to the physician in ever-expanding volume from a variety of sources, some of which are far from objective, and many of which draw contradictory conclusions. An additional problem for doctor and patient is the fact that until very recently most studies in scientific literature were directed at what is essentially the tip of the iceberg. That is, the vast majority of reports about drugs and pregnancy dealt with death and gross physical abnormalities of the fetus and newborn. Although these traditional indicators are obviously of critical importance in judging the effects of drugs, it is becoming more and more apparent that many, many substances also have to be considered in terms of their more subtle physical, neurological, and behavioral consequences in the short and the long term. These effects, although not as devastatingly dramatic as the death of an unborn baby, can have profound and permanent effects.

The sources of information that I have used for this book include my own research, contacts with colleagues who are studying drugs and pregnancy, and a variety of scientific publications, including medical, psychological, and sociological journals, government reports and bulletins, and a variety of textbooks. These publications are available in some university, hospital, and government libraries, but it is no mean feat for a pregnant woman who is not a scientist to find the particular report that contains the answer to a specific question. Making the task even more formidable is the fact that most of this work is written with specialists as the expected readers.

This state of affairs, combined with the pregnant woman's obvious need for accurate, up-to-date information, provided the impetus for this book. It is written so that the reader needs neither scientific knowledge nor familiarity with jargon to understand and assess the material covered.

To keep the text easy to read, I have included a minimum of references and usually not identified my sources of information or the authors of research studies.

The end of the book, however, suggests further reading on the topics considered in each chapter. These lists are only signposts: they are not a complete bibliography of all the material that exists on a particular matter, nor do they include all the material that was used in the preparation of this book. The references can serve, however, as a basic reading list for the reader who wishes to pursue a particular question.

THE MEANING OF PROBABILITY AND RISK

A point must be made about probability and the interpretation of scientific data. If you bet at a horserace, what you are actually doing is guessing, with a certain probability in mind, that a particular horse is going to win. Even if you place your bet on the favorite, you may lose your money because that horse may come in dead last. That the favorite doesn't always win emphasizes the fact that probability is usually not the same as a sure thing. The odds for a particular animal are designated on the basis of observations of its previous performances. The likelihood of its winning can be expressed as a probability ranging from zero to one (or 100 percent). If a horse has never won in the past and is certain never to win in the future, then the probability of its winning is zero. On the other hand, if the horse were absolutely sure to cross the finish line first, the probability of its winning would be expressed as one. Obviously, certainties—that is, probabilities of zero (a sure loser) and one (a sure winner)—don't exist in horse racing. Rather, each animal has a probability of winning that lies somewhere in between the extremes.

The interpretation of the results of scientific investigations is similar. One thing (for example, a particular drug) is rarely associated with another (for example, a specific effect in offspring) with a probability of either zero (never occurs) or one (always occurs). Rather, the relationship nearly always has a probability that falls between the two extremes.

Let's look at a specific example. Some researchers believe that drinking at alcoholic levels during pregnancy is associated with a 0.40 probability—or a 40 percent chance—of mental retardation in the offspring. In the jargon of the medical profession, this figure is called the risk factor. So the risk factor for mental retardation among the children of female alcoholics is 0.40. Knowing this risk factor enables one to have a fair idea of the likelihood of an alcoholic woman's having a mentally retarded baby compared to the chances for a mother-to-be who doesn't drink excessively but is similar to the alcoholic in all other respects.

Notice that knowing the risk factor, like knowing the odds at the race track, enables one to make only an educated prediction (some might say an educated guess), not a statement of what will happen. Certainly, predictions based on the risk factor are more likely to be right than random guesses. But exceptions will always occur. How frequently exceptions will occur—conversely, how much confidence one ought to have in educated predictions— depends on how consistently the effect in question has been found in the studies on which the risk factor is based. The more consistently the effect has been found in the past, the greater the probability of observing it in the future and the fewer the exceptions.

Understanding the meaning of probability—the degree of certainty or predictability—plays a vital role in understanding the relationship between scientific reports and the practical, real world. For example, you may read in the newspaper that a researcher has found an association between alcoholism and mental retardation. Your first reaction may be skepticism because you have a neighbor who drank like a fish while she was pregnant yet had a baby who looks and acts perfectly fine. What you have to remember is the notion of probability. Some babies will not show an adverse effect from maternal alcoholism, but the risk was still there. Most important, the absence of effect in one case does not decrease the risk in another. When one alcoholic bears a normal child, the risk factor is unchanged for a baby born to some other alcoholic woman. Thus, although the risk factor does not represent a certainty, knowing it is of critical importance for a woman who must decide whether to change her drinking habits for the sake of her unborn child.

THE SHAPE OF THIS BOOK

A necessary but often overlooked starting point for understanding how drugs may or may not affect a pregnancy is a general knowledge of how the unborn infant develops. For that reason, the first chapter of this book is a brief description of the growth of the embryo and fetus. It emphasizes the timing of the development of various structures and systems because the effect of many substances is critically dependent upon when the unborn baby is exposed to them. Also in this chapter is a discussion of the role of the placenta—the structure that transfers substances between mother and child. Can it serve as a protective barrier? The last part of the chapter is devoted to the fascinating topic of what can be revealed by physical and neurological examinations of a newborn baby and how these tests are carried out.

Having discussed the normal course of development, the book then deals with alcohol, the first of the drugs that have become incorporated into the modern life-style. Of course, drinking behavior varies widely. To keep matters in a proper perspective, separate chapters deal with the consequences of alcoholism and of social drinking during pregnancy.

Caffeine, the subject of the next chapter, is the most widely consumed stimulant drug. Yet in spite of (or perhaps because of) its ubiquitous presence, most people do not consider it a drug in beverages. In the past few years, however, the use of caffeine during pregnancy has become a very controversial issue in scientific circles.

Cigarettes and their constituents are considered next. About one baby in three is exposed to the effects of cigarettes during fetal development. The importance of knowing the consequences of this exposure is emphasized by government statistics that indicate that smoking is decreasing among all population groups save one—women of child-bearing age.

The following portion of the book deals with marijuana. As this drug is an illegal substance, it is not surprising that its use is considerably less extensive than that of alcohol, caffeine, and nicotine. However, a significant and growing number of young people "smoke up" on a fairly regular basis. The consequences of doing so during pregnancy are just now coming under scientific scrutiny.

The average household contains more than 20 over-the-counter drugs, and many pregnant women swallow them with very little thought. The final chapter deals with some of the most common of these drugs, including painkillers, cold remedies and vitamin supplements, as well as with tranquilizers, one of the most common categories of prescription drugs.

Together, the chapters in this book are built upon the premise that motherhood starts from conception, not from birth. It is neither realistic nor scientifically supportable to ask you as an expectant mother to adopt an ascetic life-style, but knowing the potential effects of some widely used substances can help you decide whether some of your habits need changing.

1   The fetus and the newborn baby

DEVELOPMENT IN THE WOMB

Like all animals, humans grow in one of two ways: their cells increase in number, or their existing cells increase in size. This is true whether one is considering the growth of the newly fertilized egg, the growth of the embryo, the development of various organs in the fetus, or the growth of the infant after birth.

At conception, a single sperm, from the approximately 350 million the male released in one ejaculation, pierces the outermost membrane of an egg, or ovum, produced by one of the woman's ovaries. Once the egg is thus fertilized, the membrane becomes impermeable to any other sperm. Since the fertilized ovum contain genes from each parent, it has, even at this earliest stage, its full hereditary background from both the mother and the father.

Within a few hours of fertilization, the single-cell ovum divides into two, which then divide and redivide. During these divisions, each new cell carries a complete replica of all the genetic material that was in the original fertilized egg.

While this cell-splitting is proceeding, the whole microscopic ball is swept down the fallopian tube (the passageway in which fertilization takes place and which connects the ovary to the uterus) and within a week reaches the uterus. For the first 24 hours there, it remains unattached in a free-floating state.

Then things rapidly change. Under the influence of hormones released by the ovaries, the inner lining of the uterus has prepared itself to receive the fertilized egg by becoming thickened and spongy. Approximately eight days after fertilization, the ovum proceeds to burrow its way into this lining. The developing egg must now start to obtain nourishment from the mother. For this reason, the cells that form the outer layer of the embryo (as the baby is called during the first six to eight weeks of life within the uterus) develop a remarkable, specialized function. They make contact with small, blood-filled spaces in the uterus, draw out substances from the maternal blood, and pass them along to the other cells of the embryo. Here then is a primitive placenta—a structure that begins its work as early as eleven days after the ovary released a single cell. For the next 36 weeks or so, the baby will depend upon the oxygen and food it obtains from the mother's blood.

Once the ovum is implanted in the uterus, the embryo's development proceeds at a phenomenally fast rate. During the first six weeks or so, cells continue to multiply and simultaneously to develop the specialization that makes it possible for them to form structures as different as bone, blood, and tissue.

During this period, one can observe the embryo's very first movements—the beating of its heart. The entire embryo is only about a quarter-inch long—less than half the diameter of a dime—when this activity starts. You can imagine how small the heart must be! Remarkably, the heart begins to beat when the embryo is only three weeks old—before the mother usually even knows that she is pregnant. This early start gives the developing heart a preeminant position in the embryonic stage. In fact, at five weeks the bright red heart is only slightly smaller than the head, and each beat shakes the entire embryo.

Only after the heart begins to function does the nervous system start to develop. Following come the beginnings of the limbs and muscles. At six weeks the human embryo appears much like the developing young of other animals, such as rats, but by the end of the first trimester (three months after conception), an amazing transition has occurred. A single cell that was far too small to be seen by the naked eye has metamorphized into a creature that is approximately three inches long, weighs about one ounce, is easily recognizable as a small human being, and has all the essential organs present and functioning in a primitive fashion.

After the first trimester, the baby—now called a fetus, from the Latin word meaning "offspring" or "young one"—continues to increase in size. Meanwhile its organs mature and begin to integrate their functions, and other changes occur that will enable it to survive the radical change from the fluid environment of the uterus to relatively independent life in air. This is the time of most rapid growth for most limbs and organs. During no other stage of life will they grow so quickly. From the third month until just before birth, fetal weight increases nearly 500-fold. The magnitude of this growth spurt is dramatically illustrated by the fact that if its speed continued into adolescence, the average teenager would be 75 feet tall and weigh several tons!

The Development of Various Systems

Importantly, different parts of the body grow at different rates during pregnancy. In part, need appears to dictate the differences. For example, the embryo's arms and legs, which are of no use inside the womb, have a relatively poor blood supply and are quite puny compared to the rest of the body. Even during the first few months after birth, when babies do not use their limbs to support their weight, the growth of arms and legs is relatively slow.

In contrast are the head and brain. The developing embryo looks big-headed as early as six weeks because certain components of the brain grow sooner and faster than the rest of the body. Remarkably, a fetus at the end of the second trimester has the same number of nerve cells as an adult. However, they are not yet fully developed. In the mature human being, these nerve cells, or neurons, which are the basic units of the nervous system, have long, branching processes that are essential for the communication of information from one nerve cell to the next. At the end of the second trimester, the fetus does not yet have these communication processes. For the remainder of the pregnancy, therefore, the neurons no longer increase in number, but the existing ones enlarge and develop, creating neuronal processes and connections. The nonneuronal cells that support and protect the nerve cells also increase tremendously. The combination of the elaboration of the existing neurons and the multiplication of the support cells results in such a dramatic increase in brain size and weight that this period is called the brain growth spurt. It lasts from the end of the second trimester until several years after birth.

The timing of the maximum growth of particular organs has important ramifications. It is during the period of rapid growth that organs are most vulnerable to the harmful effects of outside agents. Once a fetal organ has been properly formed, it is quite unlikely to be malformed no matter what happens to the mother or the fetus. Malformations that are present at birth and that have environmental causes (as opposed to genetic causes) are almost always the result of harmful influences during the first trimester. That is why, for example, it is so important to avoid exposure to the German measles virus during the first trimester and why thalidomide had its devastating effects only when it was taken early in pregnancy.

The brain, because of its almost two-stage development, is particularly vulnerable at different times. Anything that affects the brain growth spurt has potential ramifications for the establishment of neural connections and the formation of the support cells. It will not, however, have a marked effect upon the number of nerve cells as their production occurred early in pregnancy. Alterations in the brain's gross features, such as brain weight and the thickness of certain layers of cells, may result from environmental factors encountered early in pregnancy (affecting the number of neurons) or from those encountered late in pregnancy or even after birth (affecting the neuronal processes, the nerve cell connections, and the number and size of support cells).

Since the fetus spends the second and third trimesters growing, maturing, and integrating the various systems, exposure to harmful external agents at this time will have results quite different from those of exposure early in pregnancy. Whereas malformations of organs and systems are first-trimester consequences of embryonic vulnerability, perturbances during the last two trimesters are likely to alter the growth and/or function of the various structures in the fetus.

PROTECTIVE SYSTEMS

Of course, it is not only the fetus that undergoes remarkable growth and changes during pregnancy. Several specialized systems that are not actually part of the baby are necessary for the survival and development of the embryo and fetus.

The Placenta

Perhaps the most obvious of the protective systems developed during pregnancy is the placenta, which starts to function before the embryo is two weeks old and grows rapidly throughout gestation. By about the eighth month, its growth by cell division stops, but the existing cells continue to increase in size. During the approximately 280 days of pregnancy, the placenta grows from a single layer of cells to an organ that measures one inch in thickness and seven inches in diameter and that weighs an average of slightly more than a pound. At birth, it appears flat and spongy. (Appropriately, the word "placenta" derives from the Latin word for pancake).

The placenta is located in the portion of the uterus that has the most abundant blood supply. One side of the placenta is in contact with the wall of the uterus, and the other side is in contact with the fetus. On the uterine side of the primitive placenta, small fingerlike projections known as villi burrow into the lining of the uterus, where they lie bathed in small pools of blood. These villi continue to grow and branch profusely; in them develop blood vessels that connect to the fetus's circulatory system and form the umbilical cord. At one end of the umbilical cord is the embryo, and at the other is the placenta. All this within four weeks after conception! With time the villi continue to branch, providing a larger and larger area of contact between mother and baby and also a firmer and firmer attachment of the embryo to the wall of the uterus.

These anatomical developments result in the circulation of maternal blood on the outside of the placental villi and of the baby's blood on the inner surface. Under normal circumstances the two circulations never mix: the blood of the mother does not enter the fetus, nor does that of the fetus enter the mother's bloodstream. The transfer of nourishment to the fetus and of waste products to the mother takes place across the thin walls of the tiny villi of the placenta. Each time the mother's heart beats, blood loaded with oxygen and nutrients enters the pool surrounding the villi and blood loaded with carbon dioxide and waste products leaves. The pumping of the fetal heart moves the baby's blood containing waste products down one of two arteries in the umbilical cord to the placenta, where it filters across the villi. From the placenta via an umbilical vein, the fetal heart also receives blood rich in oxygen and nutritional components that have diffused from the mother's blood.

In addition to transferring nourishment and waste products between mother and child, the placenta acts as a busy, complex factory. It takes substances from both the mother and baby and, with the aid of some 60 different enzymes that it manufactures, breaks them into simpler compounds with which it manufactures new products that are appropriately redistributed to the fetus and the mother. Thus, the placenta acts like many different organs that come into complete operation only after birth. In the uterus, it functions in place of the infant's lungs (exchange of oxygen and carbon dioxide), liver (conversion of materials), and kidneys (elimination of waste products).

When physicians first realized the way in which the placenta separates the baby's blood from the mother's, they adopted the term "placental barrier." But clearly, many things do cross the placenta. It is not able to judge which of these substances may be harmful to the fetus. Whether a substance does or does not cross is not based on its advantage or disadvantage to the fetus. Rather, the controlling factor is its molecular size. Generally, the smaller the molecule, the easier and more rapid its passage across the placenta. Large molecules may be blocked or, in certain cases, so slowed that they have little physiological effect. Of particular relevance to this book is the fact that most drugs, including alcohol, are composed of small molecules and pass the placenta readily.

Thus, "placental barrier" is somewhat of a misnomer. The placenta usually does not obstruct the passage of substances but merely controls the rate of transfer according to the physical makeup of their constituents. Anything that circulates in the mother's bloodstream may cross the placenta and reach the fetus.

The Amniotic Fluid

A second system that has a role in protecting the fetus is the liquid that surrounds the fetus within the uterus. This amniotic fluid is contained within the amniotic sac, which, in turn, lies in the uterus and contains the fetus. The amniotic fluid, produced primarily by the fetus, increases in volume as the baby gets larger. During the first trimester, the embryo's skin is porous, and the amniotic fluid is thought to pass through it. As the baby grows, this permeability decreases until it disappears at about 16 weeks. From that time, the kidneys of the fetus produce a dilute urine, which becomes the main source of the fluid.

The functions of the amniotic fluid are numerous. It provides an environment of constant temperature that permits growth and movement. It serves as a buffer against shock. It inhibits the growth of certain bacteria and thereby guards against infection.

The amniotic fluid is also helpful to physicians. Samples of it can be taken and tested to determine fetal health. Since the liquid contains cells shed by the growing fetus, they, as well as the fluid itself, can be examined for signs of congenital abnormalities.

THE INFANT AT BIRTH

In considering the health of an infant at birth, doctors use several key indicators, including birth weight, the length of the pregnancy, and the functioning of physical and neurological systems as the child encounters the relatively harsh environment of the outside world.

Birth Weight

The first two and a half months of a typical pregnancy see only a small maternal weight gain—about one and one-half pounds—primarily from the growth of the uterus and an increase in the mother's blood volume. These physiological adjustments, coupled with the deposition of maternal stores of nutrients, occur at their maximum rate a few weeks before the fetus and placenta start growing at their fastest rate. Thus, an increased amount of blood is available when needed for the uterus and placenta, and an added supply of nutrients can serve the demands of the developing baby, who weighs less than an ounce at this stage. By late pregnancy, however, the fetus has become the major contributor to the overall weight gain.

Newborns who weigh six pounds three ounces to eight pounds are regarded as of "normal" birth weight. The greatest influence on birth weight is genetic factors from the mother (surprisingly, the father's genetic contribution here is negligible). Other factors known to influence birth weight include the mother's weight gain during pregnancy, placental problems, and the use of certain drugs during pregnancy.

The evidence is conflicting as to whether the human fetus can protect itself and maintain normal growth when the mother's nutritional intake is less than optimal. Some researchers argue that the baby will take from its mother's system what it needs, even if the mother can ill afford it. A classic example is what happens when a woman is not consuming enough iron: she becomes severely anemic as pregnancy progresses, yet the baby will not exhibit this syndrome. What happens is that the fetus removes the iron from the mother at the expense of her health. A further example: during World War II, women living in cities that were suffering serious food shortages bore babies who were only slightly underweight at birth.

On the other hand, the idea that the fetus can protect itself from maternal malnutrition may have to be qualified. Evidence suggests that a baby will have a close-to-normal birth weight in the face of inadequate maternal food intake only if the mother has had a previous chance to build up her own body's stores of nutrients. If her body stores are small, her level of food intake is critical in maintaining normal fetal growth. The first biological priority of the undernourished pregnant woman, according to this evidence, may be maintaining her own stores of nutrients rather than sustaining fetal growth.

Whether nature gives the fetus or the mother-to-be priority, an order of importance clearly exists within the developing fetus. In cases of extreme malnourishment, the last system to receive insufficient nutrients is the developing brain. It is this "brain-sparing" that causes babies born during famines to have disproportionately large heads at birth.

Studies investigating factors that may influence fetal development pay a lot of attention to birth weight because this measurement is considered quite an accurate indicator of prenatal well-being and a good predictor of infant mortality. For infants with birth weights of less than 3.5 pounds, the death rate is approximately 45 percent. It decreases rapidly as the birth weight approaches the normal range, then rises again for babies who weigh more than 8.75 pounds.

In medical terms, a low birth weight is less than 5.5 pounds at birth. About two-thirds of all neonatal deaths occur in the relatively small group defined by this cutoff point. Moreover, the rate of hospitalization in the first two years of life is twice as large for this group as for infants of "normal" birth weight.

Premature and Small-for-Dates Babies

The average length of pregnancy is calculated as 280 days (40 weeks) after the first day of the last normal menstrual period (although fertilization actually takes place about two weeks after the period ends). A pregnancy of anything between 37 and 42 weeks is considered normal, and the infant born at its end is called a term infant.

Only about 7 percent of all babies are born prematurely, but the majority of deaths at or near birth occur among this group. The more premature the baby, the greater the risk for serious difficulties.

The premature infant looks skinny and is usually pinkish red because layers of fat have not had a chance to develop and blood vessels show through the thin skin. The paucity of fat also means that these babies are less capable than most of insulating themselves and are very vulnerable to cold. Because their muscles lack development, they tend to be floppy and to lie in a sprawled rather than a curled or "fetal" position. The creases and lines that a full-term baby has on its palms and soles and the complex folds of the ears are not as pronounced in the premature infant, making this baby look relatively smooth skinned.

Prematurity is associated with a number of problems in newborns. The immaturity of the lungs can result in respiratory distress, and the immaturity of the liver in severe jaundice. The softer-than-normal bones of the skull may be unable to protect the immature brain from the compression of the head that occurs during labor and delivery. These are some of the reasons that disproportionately more premature babies than full-term babies die in early infancy or suffer serious handicaps, such as cerebral palsey or mental deficiency. However, most premature babies turn out fine, both mentally and physically, and by age two and a half are indistinguishable from term babies.

Preterm babies are usually smaller than term babies, but they are an appropriate size for the length of time they have been in the uterus. A second group of babies are born small but for a different reason—they have grown too slowly in the uterus, usually because they did not get enough nourishment via the placenta. These babies, who are not necessarily premature, are described as small-for-dates as they are smaller than normal for the time they have been carried.

Only in size do small-for-dates babies resemble premature infants. Small-for-dates babies are thin and have loose flesh that give them the appearance of having recently lost weight. Because of "brain sparing," the head may seem large in proportion to the rest of the body. Overall, these infants have fewer problems at birth than premature babies.

Like preterm babies, small-for-dates babies exhibit a marked catch-up in the first 18 months of life, but then the catch-up process stops. As a consequence, unlike most children born preterm, small-for-dates children tend to be shorter and lighter than their peers even at five years of age.

Presentation for Delivery

During the third trimester, the size of the fetus leaves it little room to maneuver within the uterus, so it tends to take the most comfortable position possible—lying with its spine parallel to its mother's. Although most animals are born feet first, humans are not. By the end of the third trimester, 96 percent of babies are head down in the uterus. Breech presentations, in which the baby is not lying upside down and thus the buttocks are presented for delivery first, are relatively more frequent among premature babies and the second of a pair of twins. Because of the problems during labor that often accompany breech births, more than half of these infants are delivered by cesarean section.

Changes at Birth

The major impact of birth is the sudden, dramatic change in environment. In the womb, the baby has lived in a world of darkness with the loud constant noise of the surgings of the mother's blood, comfortably and securely supported in the warm bath of amniotic fluid. It has flailed its arms, kicked its legs, moved its chest in and out in pseudobreathing, passed urine, and may have sucked its thumb. Despite all these miraculous developments, the baby has been an essentially passive entity, entirely dependent on the transfer of supplies and wastes via the placenta. At birth, the shift in environment sets in motion a wide variety of adaptive changes ranging from new bodily functions, such as breathing and feeding, to adjusting to the multitude of new stimuli received by the sense organs. The lungs fill with air instead of the amniotic fluid, the skin is no longer surrounded by its liquid covering, and the arms and legs can move much more freely. The background sound level is reduced, but there are now many more sudden, nonrepetitive noises. The light level is increased, as is the complexity of the visual stimuli. The surrounding temperature falls and is not as constant. The typical baby loses about 6 to 9 percent of its body weight during the first four days and usually does not reach its birth weight again until just over a week.

The tight squeeze that occurred during normal vaginal delivery is evidenced by the molding of the head into a slightly more narrow and elongated shape than is seen in older babies. (The brain is, at this stage, flexible enough to accommodate this temporary change.) This molding does not occur in babies born by cesarean section and is different in breech babies, whose heads passed through the birth canal last and comparatively quickly.

Immediately after birth the baby must breathe, and those first few breaths represent very hard work. In the womb, the lungs, nose, and mouth are full of fluid. During delivery, this fluid drains out of the mouth and nose, and the squeezing of the chest forces some of the fluid from the lungs. In spite of this partial draining, some liquid remains. Coupled with this handicap is the effort needed to draw air into lungs that are totally devoid of air—a much greater effort than is required to inhale air into lungs that already contain some. After the first few gasps, the lungs become partially expanded, and subsequent breathing becomes easier and easier. A healthy baby takes a few days to achieve full expansion of the lungs. Some premature babies have lungs too immature to be capable of holding air after expiration, so each inhalation involves drawing air into a collapsed lung and requires enormous effort. Continued effort of this nature results in exhaustion and respiratory distress.

Concurrent with the first few breaths are changes in the baby's circulatory system, the most dramatic to occur at birth. In utero, the placenta provided oxygen and removed carbon dioxide; since the lungs were not being used for breathing, little blood was directed toward them. At birth, of course, this all changes. The placenta becomes detached from the uterus and is passed out the vagina as the afterbirth. The arteries that carried blood from the baby to the placenta via the umbilical cord constrict and close, and the blood flow to the baby's lungs increases. In addition, a hole in the wall between two chambers of the heart is blocked. In the uterus, the fetus's heart pumped blood to its body and the placenta and then back to the heart. Now it has to go first through the lungs where it picks up oxygen and deposits waste gases, such as carbon dioxide. It is the closing of the hole in the heart that forces the blood to take the heart-lungs-heart-body circuit. These remarkable changes all occur as a healthy baby takes its first few breaths.

The loss of the attachment to the placenta also means that the baby is cut off from its source of automatic nourishment. Until the first feeding, the baby must rely on nutrients stored in the liver. Babies who are either premature or small-for-dates may not have a sufficient reserve and so require special care.

The Apgar Test at Birth

Some babies cry immediately after birth, whereas others do not make a sound. However, most start to move their arms and legs very soon. Doctors look for this movement as one of the signs of a healthy baby.

Most hospitals make a quick examination for these and other signs of health at one and five minutes after birth. This procedure, termed the Apgar test, uses five parameters: heart rate, respiratory effort, muscular tone, reflex responses, and color. The baby is rated on each item using a scale of zero to two; the points are added together, making ten the maximum score. For example, a baby with a blue-white color scores zero for that parameter; a pink body and the blue extremities merit one point; a completely pink baby gets two points. Most babies get a total score of seven to ten in each Apgar test session. A score of four to six usually indicates the presence of mild to moderate breathing difficulties. A newborn is considered severely depressed and in danger when the Apgar score is two or less.

These examinations during the first few minutes of life are quick procedures to assess the newborn's ability to cope with the stress of labor, delivery, and adjustment to the outside world. Useful as the Apgar test is, it is limited to providing a measure of the infant's capacity for the first five minutes of life only. It does not serve as a good predictor of how the infant will do later on.

THE FIRST FEW DAYS

The newborn is a contradiction. The baby appears totally helpless yet is extraordinarily good at a number of things. The new baby is a specialist but more open to change than he or she will ever be again. During the first few days the baby fluctuates repeatedly between sleep and wakefulness with considerable apparent irritability during the waking hours. Hiccups, tremors, uncoordinated eye movements, irregular breathing, and oscillations in body temperature and skin color indicate that the internal regulation of the newborn has not quite stabilized. After a few days many of these irregularities disappear as the baby begins to adapt to the extraordinary change of environment.

What Doctors Look For

Considerable importance is placed upon the physical appearance of the newborn's external features because they are useful indicators of whether normal development has taken place in the uterus. Characteristics of the skin, hands, feet, eyes, and ears can all be used for this purpose. For example, an abnormal slant or an unusual distance between the eyes, an extra finger or toe, or ears that are located somewhat lower than usual may be subtle signals of abnormal development. Doctors give such signs considerable significance neither for aesthetic reasons nor in the belief that an unusual appearance prevents normal function. Rather, when structural abnormalities are present, the chances of the nervous system not having developed normally increase considerably. It is as if unusual external features signal the possibility of more hidden and possibly more serious abnormalities. In a similar fashion, when physical growth is not normal for the length of gestation, the factors that caused underdevelopment of size may also have resulted in immaturity of the nervous system.

Because of the fluctuations in the baby's systems during the first few days of its life plus the possible aftereffects of the birth process and any anesthetics and analgesics used during labor, the first examination of the newborn's behavior is usually postponed until several days after the birth.

The Newborn's Response to Stimuli

Although the infant of less than a week old is helpless and dependent on others, it is quite wrong to think of the newborn as a blank slate. Lying in a tiny bassinet, the baby makes seemingly random movements that may suggest no behavioral repertoire, no likes and dislikes, no adaptive or self-controlling abilities, and no social responsiveness. Not true! In fact, some kinds of behavior started or had their origin before birth. First, the genetic endowment present from conception may predispose the fetus to certain kinds of behavior, such as a particular level of activity or reflection of temperament.

In addition, the fetus has gained experience from the later part of the nine-month stay in the mother's uterus.

Many a women can attest to the fact that the active and quiet times of her baby during pregnancy became associated with her own rest, sleep, and activity cycles. Perhaps more startling is the fact that experiments have shown that babies can hear and see in the uterus. A loud, sudden noise applied next to the abdomen can cause the fetus to startle. At a gentle, soft sound, the fetus may move and turn slowly toward the noise. In a parallel fashion, a flash of a bright white light directed at the fetus's line of vision can cause a startle reaction. These findings certainly lend credence to the idea that different types of music may affect an unborn baby and that the effect is a direct one rather than a phenomenon based on some response of the mother's being relayed to the baby.

It was long a basic premise that the newborn's world was, as described so picturesquely by William James, the eminent 19th-century American psychologist, as a "blooming, buzzing confusion." The idea was that the sense organs, in particular those of vision and hearing, were so poorly developed at birth as to be virtually useless. Modern evidence now clearly indicates that, in fact, even the very young baby can make some sense of the environment and can learn from experience.

The newborn comes into the outside world equipped with quite a large array of reflexes that serve as self-protection, facilitate the finding and obtaining of food, and enhance the seeking of stimulation. A number of these reflexes also form the basis of complex, coordinated voluntary movements of later childhood.

The movements that the baby makes during the first days and weeks of life are not, despite appearances to the contrary, without purpose. Healthy newborns respond to stimulation. They also show distinct likes and dislikes—and the existence of preferences means, of course, that they can discriminate among stimuli. Take hearing, for example. Newborns are sensitive to a wide range of sounds and turn in response to them, showing the ability to locate the direction of their source. Babies shows a preference for high-pitched rather than low-pitched sounds and react most positively, in terms of attention, to the human voice.

Visually, neonates also seem to prefer certain objects. For example, when a shiny red ball is held about ten inches in front of a newborn's eyes, the eyes widen, the head and neck move slightly, and the arms and legs relax. Balls of other, duller colors are not as attractive. Remarkably, the most attractive visual stimulus in terms of keeping a neonate's attention is the human face. Even a life-size cutout picture of a face works. Thus, the very young baby's ears and eyes both have a special sensitivity to stimuli that are the most essential for survival and socialization—stimuli that are usually provided by the parents' natural actions.

Within a few days of birth, the baby's eyes can follow moving objects and, within a month, can focus on objects as much as a few feet away. Ten inches appears to be the best distance for the newborn. Targets that are jiggled about this distance in front of the baby and then moved back and forth slowly are "caught" and followed by the eyes, and, on occasion, even the head may turn to follow the image. It is easy to see how all these factors are conducive to bonding in the natural situation of a mother's breast-feeding and quietly talking to her baby.

Habituation and the Brazelton Scale

Not only can newborns respond differentially to different stimuli; they can also shut out and seemingly ignore some forms of stimulation. This ability is of enormous importance. As soon as the baby enters the world, the sensory systems are exposed to a veritable bombardment of stimuli, many of which are of little relevance to the infant. Other stimuli, if continuously reacted to, would make too many demands on the baby's energy.

Not responding to input is vividly seen in a recently developed test designed to examine the newborn's capacity to interact with the environment. The procedures, devised by Terry Brazelton, a Boston pediatrician, are part of the Brazelton Neonatal Assessment Scale, which was first described in 1973 and is now used in more than 200 hospitals and research facilities to examine the newborn's relationship with the outside world.

The Brazelton tests administered to babies at about four days of age examine the ability to shut out stimuli in a variety of ways. One procedure consists of shaking a fairly loud rattle for one or two seconds near the ear of a baby who is partially awake. The infant's reaction is similar to yours or mine. It is a startle response in which all four limbs move vigorously, the eyes blink open (or possibly squeeze tightly closed), and the rate of breathing increases. If the rattle noise is repeated approximately every five seconds, the first few shakes continue to elicit startles, but they gradually diminish. In most infants, the vigor of the startle is noticeably less after the fifth or sixth shake, and by the eighth or ninth many have ceased responding at all and revert to their initial drowsy state. The same shutdown can be seen if the sudden sound is replaced by a light flashed at the eyes while they are lightly closed. The first few flashes result in vigorous startles, but a gradual shutdown occurs if the presentations are continued.

This diminution in responsiveness to repeated stimuli is termed habituation. It is a complex process thought to reflect a maturing, healthy nervous system. Habituation has the purpose of helping the newborn baby both cope with a surfeit of stimulation and conserve the relatively limited amount of available energy by diminishing the extent of the startle response.

This latter property of habituation is dramatically shown in another Brazelton test that involves pricking the baby's foot lightly with a pin. The reaction the first time is quite predictable. A startle occurs, and both feet are withdrawn; fussing and vigorous movements of the arms and legs follow. When the pinpricks are repeated, however, most infants reduce their responses remarkably, so that the seventh or eighth elicts only a pushing-away motion with one foot. Only the essential component of the response remains, minimizing the amount of energy used.

Habituation is a coping response. If it fails, one consequence is considerable agitation, which, quite naturally, results in exhaustion and irritability. Babies who have difficulty in habituation may, therefore, spend an unusually large amount of their time sleeping and crying. One result of both kinds of behavior is the shutting out of stimuli from the seemingly unfriendly new world.

Habituation is not by any means the only self-protective mechanism at the healthy newborn's disposal. For example, if a piece of light cloth is placed over the face, the typical baby goes through a series of movements to remove it. The first reaction is usually movement of the mouth. If this doesn't move the offending stimulus, the head is turned from side to side. Finally, if the cloth still remains, swiping motions with the hands are directed at it.

Movement and Neurological Development

The series of defensive reactions that serve to keep the eyes and face clear also provide evidence of the nervous system's muscular control. In general, movement can tell quite a bit about whether the newborn's nervous system has developed normally. The spontaneous movements of the limbs are important in this respect. For example, all babies make fists, but some infants who have had fetal difficulties, such as a deficiency of oxygen, do not unclench their hands even when relaxed. Again, a healthy full-term baby frequently lies with arms and legs in a flexed position and the tone in the flexor muscles is quite marked. Even the muscles controlling the movement of the head show some degree of control in the first days. If one holds a healthy full-term newborn face downward, supporting the stomach and chest, the baby lifts his head, thereby exhibiting the very early signs of postural control.

One of the most important ways of testing the integrity

of the nervous system is the examination of the reflexes that form so much of the newborn's behavioral repertoire. For example, a stepping reflex can be seen within a few days of birth. It can be elicited by holding the baby upright, leaning forward slightly with the feet in contact with a firm surface. The result is usually a jerky, high-stepping movement that is a useful test of the ability to move the legs in an integrated fashion. This reflex starts to disappear at three to four weeks of age.

The Mora reflex offers a way to check the movements of the arms. It is set off by a sudden motion that gives the baby a feeling of falling. The startle that this evokes results in a flinging out of the arms, a spreading of the hands, and often a cry. Then the infant begins to close the hands and bring the arms back together, seemingly to clasp anyone or anything within reach.

The coordination of movements in other parts of the body can be observed by eliciting other reflexes. For example, a gentle touch on one of the baby's cheeks results in the rooting reflex—a turning of the head toward the side that was touched. Functionally, this reflex encourages the baby to turn to the nipple when the mother's breast touches the cheek. Once a stimulus, such as the nipple, touches the mouth, a sucking reflex usually ensues. Coordination of the fingers can be seen in the grasp reflex, which can be set off by gently touching the baby's palm with one's thumb. The infant curls his fingers around and grips the thumb with surprising strength. Trying to pull away usually results in an increasing grasp, which is frequently strong enough to enable the baby to be lifted up by the grip of the two hands.

The manner in which the reflexes are performed and their strength are useful signs of the way in which the nervous system is functioning. Neurological abnormalities may prevent normal, smooth reflex movements or may result in unusual or exaggerated responses or an undue number of startles and tremors.

Learning in the Newborn

Reflexes have also been used to provide convincing evidence that the newborn baby, far from being a "blooming, buzzing confusion," is quite aware of much of the surroundings and can even learn from them. One such study used the rooting response of babies two to six days old. The infants, while lying on their backs, had their cheeks stroked while a tone was sounded. If the babies turned their heads in the appropriate direction, they were rewarded by being allowed to suck on nipples. At the outset, the babies turned in response to the tone alone (without their cheeks' being touched) an average of 25 percent of the time. After half an hour of "training," they turned at the tone 75 percent of the time. Clearly, they had learned to associate the sound with the reward of being allowed to suckle.

The experiment continued with a further twist. A different tone was introduced when the cheeks were stroked, but no reward was given if the babies turned their heads. They continued to get rewarded, however, when they turned in response to the original tone. Within 30 minutes of this two-tone training, the infants demonstrated a clear ability to discriminate. When the "correct" tone was sounded without any cheek stroking, head turns continued to occur on about 75 percent of the trials; when the "incorrect" tone sounded, the head turns stayed at the initial baseline level of 25 percent. So, not only can newborns learn to associate one event with another, but they can also learn to tell the difference between rewarded and unrewarded stimuli.

THE VULNERABLE TIME OF LIFE

This chapter has only sketched the journey from the single cell at conception to the immensely complex infant of a few days of age who is capable of learning. What makes this nine-month span so amazing is the rapidity and the scope of the development it encompasses. Unfortunately, it is the very extent and rapidity of these changes that make the developing embryo and fetus so vulnerable to environmental insults. The ways in which various drugs can have lifelong repercussions are the focus of discussion in the following chapters.

2 Alcohol: The alcoholic mother-to-be

Alcohol is as old as civilization itself. A brewery is said to have existed in Egypt 23 centuries before the dynasty of King Tutankhamen. The writings of ancient Chinese and Indian cultures from as long ago as 2000 B.C. include discussions of alcohol.

When one considers the length of time that alcohol has been associated with human societies, it is somewhat surprising that scientists have so recently discovered the interaction of alcohol and pregnancy. "Rediscovered" might be a better term. The 1970s and early 1980s saw a surge of interest in the topic, but it was scarcely a new found phenomenon.

ALCOHOL AND PREGNANCY: A LOOK AT HISTORY

One of the earliest warnings about alcohol and pregnancy can be found in the Christian bible: "'Behold, you shall conceive and bear a son; so then drink no wine or strong drink, and eat nothing unclean'" (Judges 13:7).

The bible was not the only early writing to advise on the issue of alcohol and offspring. In ancient Greece where wine was so generally used that social gatherings were called *symposia*, which means drinking together, leading philosophers suggested rules to govern drinking. For example, Plato, in approximately 350 B.C., recommended limits on the number of vineyards in any city, abstinence during daytime, no drinking at any time for boat pilots or slaves, and, particularly germaine for our topic, prohibition for parents during procreation. Plato's student Aristotle continued the last line of thought by declaring, "Foolish, drunken and hare-brained women most often bring forth children like unto themselves, morose and languid." In the second century, Plutarch, another Greek philosopher, stated, "One drunkard begets another." The ancient cities of Carthage and Sparta both had laws that prohibited a newly married couple from drinking on their wedding night so that conception would not occur during intoxication. Interestingly, in Roman mythology, Vulcan, the deformed god of fire and metal-working, was said to be the product of a drunken union.

"The Gin Epidemic" of 18th-Century London

In England during the early 1700s, a complex of social and political forces, including the land-holding aristocracy's desire to sell more grain, led to a rise in the number of distillers in the country and hence to a phenomenal increase in the amount of gin drunk. In 1685, approximately half a million gallons of gin were consumed. By 1714, the figure was 2 million. By 1742, it had leaped to more than 7 million, and by 1750, to an astounding 11 million gallons. Londoners drank most of the gin produced, and their average consumption was a staggering 10.5 gallons per person per year. In 20th-century terms that works out to more than 42 40-ounce bottles of gin for every man, woman, and child—a per-capita consumption about 700 percent greater than that of all kinds of distilled alcohol in the present-day United States.

Gin was available absolutely everywhere. In the largest parish in London, one house in five was licensed to sell it. Perhaps the very first coin-operated vending machine came into existence during this flood of alcohol. Passersby were urged to place money in the mouth of a metal cat attached to a window sill and whisper "Puss! Give me two pence worth of gin." Down a pipe would come a shot.

The effects of this deluge of gin became more and more appalling, and in 1751 the government acted to control its abuse. Consumption dropped to 2 million gallons in 1785 and to about a million by 1790.

Why did the parliament act to stop the gin epidemic? One of the key reasons was the population decline. Between 1730 and 1749, 75 percent of all children christened died before the age of five. The blame for this stark statistic was placed squarely upon gin. In 1726, the College of Physicians told parliament that gin was "a cause of weak, feeble and distempered children." Ten years later a government report found:

> With regard to the female sex, we find the [gin drinking] has spread even among them, and that to a degree hardly possible to be conceived. Unhappy mothers habituate themselves to these distilled liquors, whose children are born weak and sickly, and often look shrivel'd and old as though they had numbered years. Others again daily give it to their children and learn even before they can go, to taste and approve this certain destroyer.

Two men are generally credited with raising the public conscience about the gin laws. One was Henry Fielding, a novelist, playwright, lawyer, and chief of police of the inner part of London. The other was William Hogarth, the painter and engraver.

Henry Fielding, known today primarily as the author of *The History of Tom Jones, A Foundling*, became chief magistrate in 1748 and played a major role in controlling crime in London. His pamphlets containing observations and advice on crime and drunkenness became the basis for several reform acts of parliament. It was Fielding who, in 1751, asked the question that is still being asked more than 230 years later. In a petition entitled *An Enquiry into the Cause of the Late Increase of Robbers*, he wrote:

> What must become an infant who is conceived in Gin? with the poisonous Distillations of which it is nourished, both in the Womb and at the Breast.

Perhaps even more than Fielding, the artist William Hogarth aroused the public to such a furor that the politicians had to act. In 1751, he produced a series of realistic and inexpensive prints that provided moral lessons about contemporary social problems. *Gin Lane*, reproduced here, was a particularly strong portrayal of the effects of alcohol on children. The dominent figure is a drunken mother sitting on steps taking snuff while her baby falls over a flight of stairs onto the street below. Next to the steps is a gin shop, over its door a sign, "Drunk for a penny, dead drunk for twopence, clean straw for nothing." Above, a carpenter and housewife are pawning their possessions. (One common term for gin was "strip-me-naked.") Among the smaller figures in the print are a mother giving gin to her baby, two orphan girls in charity dresses sharing a glass of gin, and a man, driven mad by gin, who has spitted a child upon a stick. The only buildings not crumbling into ruins are the pawnshop, a distillery, and an undertaker's premises marked with a coffin.

According to historians, the picture given by this print is essentially true. The various crimes portrayed are recorded in court documents. The scene depicted was in the parish of St. Giles where at least every fourth house was a gin shop. The wide distribution of this print was an important contributing factor to the marked drop in gin sales that began in London after 1751.

Before leaving England of the mid-18th century and

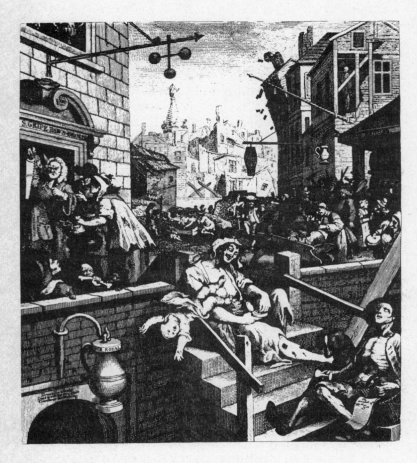

William Hogath's *Gin Lane*: London, 1751

its concern over parental gin-drinking, it is worth noting that the contemporary denunciation of that form of liquor was not an overall condemnation of alcohol. The drinking of strong beer was devoutly defended; in fact, reformers argued that one of the evil consequences of gin drinking was a decline in the consumption of beer. One has to wonder about this "decline." A 1722 estimate was that the annual per-capita consumption was 43 U.S. gallons!

Alcohol in America

Alcohol was certainly not limited to the British side of the Atlantic Ocean during the 18th century. It had been one of the facts of daily life from the very beginning of American history. Distilled spirits accompanied the colonists of Virginia in 1607. A few years later alcohol was specified in America's first drug law, which defined a drunkard as "a person that lisps or faults in his speech by reason of drink, or that staggers in his going, or that vomits or cannot follow his calling."

According to some historians, the island of Manhatten owes its name to alcohol. They claim that the word is derived from the Indian name Manahachtanienk, meaning "the place where we all got drunk." It is not clear whether this name was given because Henry Hudson brought alcohol from his boat to help in making friends with the Indians or because the Dutch payment for the island included a barrel of rum.

Whether this history of Manhatten's name is apocryphal or not, alcohol played a very visible role in America's early society. According to some, the two basic social institutions of pioneer America were the church and the tavern. The innkeeper was a man of considerable influence and merchants who dealt in alcohol were respected.

By the time Independence had been declared, the problems associated with excess drinking, although certainly not of the magnitude England had faced during the gin epidemic earlier in the century, were of concern to a number of prominent Americans. In the forefront was the physician Benjamin Rush, a signer of the Declaration of Independence. In 1776 he published the first American scientific work on alcohol abuse, *An Inquiry into the Effects of Ardent Spirits Upon the Human Body and Mind*, which was in its eighth edition by 1814.

Rush's writings are thought to have served as the impetus for the earliest American temperance societies. Modern readers find many of his statements old-fashioned and moralistic—take, for example, his Moral and Physical Thermometer, reproduced here. Nevertheless, Rush made a number of important and wise medical and social observations. He was one of the first to consider alcoholism a disease—a concept that is still being debated today. (It should be noted, however, that Rush also considered pregnancy a disease.)

In the article that included the Moral and Physical Thermometer, Rush advised against prescribing alcohol to pregnant women because of its potential for creating dependence. In the same pamphlet, in a section that described the various ways in which people were introduced to excessive drinking, he noted:

> Women have sometimes been led to seek relief from what is called breeding sickness [morning sickness], by the use of ardent spirits. A little gingerbread, or biscuit, taken occasionally, so as to prevent the stomach being empty, is a much better remedy for that disease. (Rush, 1814, pp. 2-3)

The Temperance Movement and Prohibition

In 1826, the American Temperance Society was born; by 1833, its membership was close to 300 thousand. Initially a religious movement, the Society first preached moderate drinking or temperance, later proposed abstinence and finally demanded nationwide prohibition. Although vol-

A MORAL AND PHYSICAL THERMOMETER.
A scale of the progress of Temperance and Intemperance.—Liquors with effects in their usual order.

		TEMPERANCE.
70	Water,	Health and Wealth.
60	Milk and Water,	
50	Small Beer,	Serenity of Mind, Reputation, Long Life, & Happiness.
40	Cider and Perry,	
30	Wine,	Cheerfulness, Strength, and Nourishment, when
20	Porter,	taken only in small quantities, and at meals.
10	Strong Beer,	
0		

INTEMPERANCE.

		VICES.	DISEASES.	PUNISH-MENTS.
0				
10	Punch,	Idleness, Gaming,	Sickness,	Debt.
20	Toddy and Egg Rum,	peevishness,	Tremors of the hands in the morning, puking,	Jail.
30	Grog—Brandy and Water,	quarrelling Fighting,	bloatedness, Inflamed eyes, red nose	Black eyes, and Rags,
40	Flip and Shrub,	Horse-Racing,	and face, Sore and swelled legs,	Hospital or Poor house.
50	Bitters infused in Spirits and Cordials.	Lying and Swearing,	jaundice, Pains in the hands, burn-	
60	Drams of Gin, Brandy, and Rum, in the morning,	Stealing & Swindling,	ing in the hands, and feet Dropsy, Epilepsy,	Bridewell. State prison
70	The same morning and ning. The same during day & night,	Perjury, Burglary, Murder,	Melancholy, palsy, apoplexy, Madness, Despair,	do. for Life. Gallows.

A View of Alcohol at the Time of the American Revolution

Source: Benjamin Rush, *An Inquiry into the Effects of Ardent Spirits Upon the human Body and Mind*, 8th ed. (Brookfield, Mass.: Merriam & Co., 1814), pp. 2–3, as reprinted in *Quarterly Journal of Studies on Alcohol* 4 (1943): 324.

umes were written during the first half of the 1800s on the general effects of alcohol, relatively little attention was paid to the issue of drinking and pregnancy. About the middle of the century, however, the supposed consequences of maternal drinking began to be described in vivid terms more and more frequently in order to support the philosophy of the Temperance movement. For example, in 1857 a physician warned:

> When the brain and nervous system have been the subject of such torturing persecution; at one time lashed into fury, and at another, sunk to the lowest depths of depression, is it wonderful that the offspring of such parents should inherit a weak and perverted nervous system—overthrown by the least unusual exciting cause, subject to spasms, convulsions, and falling readily into attacks of epilepsy or idiocy? Not only is this peculiarly delicate and irritable temperament transmissible from parent to child, but descends even to the third generation. (P. Stevens, 1857)

Alcohol Research in the 1940s and 1950s

During the Prohibition years of 1920 to 1933, virtually no scientific work was reported on alcohol and pregnancy, possibly because researchers thought that if alcohol were no longer sold or drunk legally, the issue was no longer relevant. Not until the 1940s was there a resurgence of interest in alcohol's effects on children and unborn babies. Paralleling contemporary society's tendency to dismiss Prohibition as a period of excessive and inappropriate moralism, medical writers and scientists did not put much stock in the pre-Prohibition era's findings on alcohol-related subjects. They argued that the research had frequently not been objective as the investigators had an antialcohol bias and were looking for data to support their point of view.

During the 1940s and 1950s, many scientists thought

that sociological and environmental factors were the key elements in producing the effects earlier workers had reported. According to this theory, an alcoholic woman might have children who were abnormal, either physically or mentally, but they were that way because the mother had received inadequate nutrition during pregnancy or because the rearing conditions in the home were so poor. Alcohol was not the direct cause. There was also a belief that mental retardation and alcoholism in the offspring of such a family were rooted in a general inheritable trait. In other words, "while alcohol does not make bad stock, many alcoholics come from bad stock."

THE DISCOVERY OF THE FETAL ALCOHOL SYNDROME

Not until the 1970s did the pendulum swing once more. The shift was the result of a major "discovery."

At a meeting of the National Council on Alcoholism in 1971, a young pediatrician from the University of Washington in Seattle reported a finding that even staid scientists considered dramatic. She had been puzzled by six infants who, in spite of good medical care, were not growing or developing normally. In tracking down the possible causes for this "failure to thrive," as medical jargon euphemistically calls it, the pediatrician made a startling disovery. The six infants all had one thing in common—each had a mother who was an alcoholic.

Persuing this apparent link between failure to·thrive and heavy alcohol consumption during pregnancy, the pediatrician reviewed hospital files from an 18-month period and managed to identify 12 babies who had been born to alcoholics. Ten of them were undersized at birth. Of the ten who had been given developmental tests, five had retarded development, three were borderline, and only two were normal. And as these ten children grew, eight continued to be much smaller than other children their age in terms of weight and head circumference.

The next part of the story took about two years to

unfold. Two physicians at the University of Washington whose speciality was the detection of birth defects examined eight of the children identified by their fellow pediatrician. Four had the same pattern of physical abnormalities. The specialists then located seven other infants who showed a similar pattern of physical anomalies. In each case, the mother had been an alcoholic during pregnancy. The doctors reported their observations on the characteristics of these eleven children in the scientific literature in 1973, calling the pattern of abnormalities the fetal alcohol syndrome—commonly abbreviated as FAS.

Ironically, these findings were summarized as "the first reported association between maternal drinking and aberrant morphogenesis in the offspring." But even if this claim was late by many decades, the identification and labeling of a recognizable pattern of features linked to prenatal exposure to alcohol did ignite an explosion of scientific activity in the area.

Teratology and the Thalidomide Tragedy

The resurgence of interest in alcohol's intrauterine effects was also encouraged by the burgeoning field of drug research termed teratology. Teratologists are scientists who examine a drug's tendency to induce abnormal development and birth defects when administered during gestation. The term is derived from the Greek word for monster, because teratology originally concentrated on physical deformities. (Not surprisingly, drugs producing such effects are called teratogens.) Today, teratology is also concerned with other alterations in the offspring, including impaired behavioral and intellectual development.

Mammalian teratology began in the 1930s, although studies on lower classes of animals had been carried out at least a century earlier. It was in the early 1960s, however, that human teratology suddenly received a great deal of attention. The reason was the thalidomide tragedy in which a mild sedative that was recommended for expectant mothers resulted in effects that are all too well known today. When taken during the fifth to seventh week of pregnancy, even single doses of the drug resulted in a baby's lacking the long bones of the arms and/or legs with the hands and/or feet close to the trunk, giving a flipper-like look to the limbs.

This tragedy provided a number of painful lessons pertinent to the alcohol issue. One of the reasons thalidomide had been prescribed was because it was thought to be so safe. No untoward effects had been noted when the drug had been given to pregnant rats. Doses 10 to 15 times the recommended level could be taken by nonpregnant adults and even children without obvious side effects.

An apparent lack of correspondence between the effects on the developing fetus and on mature individuals is a general property of most drugs that affect fetal development. Certainly, alcohol has a wide variety of toxic consequences for the adult, but they do not appear to provide the means for understanding or predicting its impact on the unborn baby.

Just as thalidomide caused a particular pattern of malformations, most other teratogenic agents also seem to produce a specific cluster of effects. However, a complete pattern is only the extreme of a spectrum of damage. Most teratogens, including alcohol, can vary considerably in the extent and severity of their impact. It is crucial to emphasize this point. Alcohol's potential effects range from very mild to very severe. The fetal alcohol syndrome is the most severe end of the spectrum, and its occurrence depends on a combination of factors, including the quantity and timing of the mother's drinking, the genetic constitution of the baby, and, possibly, the presence or absence of other nonalcohol risk factors.

To muddy the issue a little more, teratogens rarely cause abnormalities in all the fetuses that are exposed. Variations can occur in cases of the same amount and timing of the exposure. Two reports of fraternal twins born to alcoholic mothers offer a dramatic example. In each case, the two babies, arising from separate eggs with different genetic constituents yet developing in the uterus at the same time, were exposed to similar amounts of alcohol at similar stages of development. However, one twin of each pair was much more affected than the other. One showed all the characteristics associated with the fetal alcohol syndrome, whereas the other was only minimally affected. In fact, according to the pediatricians who described them, the baby who showed the lesser influence of the prenatal exposure would probably not have been identified as affected had the physicians not taken a particularly close look because of the severe problems of the other member of the twin pair. These studies emphasize the importance of genetic factors in determining the extent of alcohol's influence on the developing fetus.

CHARACTERISTICS OF THE FETAL ALCOHOL SYNDROME

What are the characteristics of infants who, in terms of live births, represent the extreme end of the spectrum of fetal problems related to the drinking of alcohol during pregnancy? In 1980, scientists, after reviewing 245 cases from many countries, including the United States, Canada, Australia, West Germany, France, South Africa, and Sweden, decided that the FAS label should be applied only on seeing symptoms in each of three categories:

1. Retardation of prenatal and/or postnatal growth, in terms of weight, length, and/or head circumference.
2. Central nervous system involvement, which may show itself as some sort of neurological abnormality, developmental delay, or intellectual deficit.
3. Particular facial features associated with the syndrome.

Let's consider each of these three in detail.

Growth Retardation

The determination of whether growth is retarded involves comparing the size of the child to information in standard growth charts. Such charts, which have been derived over the years from hospital birth records and the files of physicians, provide what can be called normative data. They give not only average length, weight, and head circumference at various ages but also the range of measurements that have been found. In order for a suspected FAS child to be considered growth-retarded, the measurement must be less than those of 90 percent of all the children whose scores make up the growth charts. In other words, theoretically, if one took 100 children of the same age, 90 of them would be taller or weigh more or have larger head circumferences than the child diagnosed as having the fetal alcohol syndrome.

The growth deficiency associated with alcohol starts during the development in the uterus but, importantly, is not overcome after birth. There is no postnatal catch-up, even when the children are reared in foster homes where they are fed more-than-adequate diets. FAS children remain smaller than 90 percent of children of the same age.

Some researchers have found that although excessive maternal drinking reduces both length and weight, weight is the more affected. They report that as such children develop, the relative amount of fatty tissue on their bodies diminishes, resulting in individuals who are often underweight for already reduced length. Consequently, as these babies progress through infancy and childhood, they often look very thin. In fact, their appearance makes them easy to misdiagnose as cases of "failing to thrive" caused by postnatal circumstances, such as inadequate feeding during the first year or two of life.

The presence of prenatal growth retardation is assessed by the baby's birth weight. As we have seen, there are two kinds of babies who are small at birth. One group is small because they are born well before the 280-day gestation period has elapsed, and they have simply not had enough time to grow. Other babies, full term or preterm, have just not grown to the degree considered normal for the length of time that they have been carried. It is these small-for-dates newborns who show the effects of intra-uterine growth deficiencies.

Alcohol is associated with the small-for-dates infants, and there is virtual unanimity in the scientific community that their low birth weight is a consequence of fetal growth retardation. It has been estimated that alcohol, in the quantities drunk by mothers who abuse it, doubles the risk factor for unusually small babies.

Unfortunately, for most women who are alcoholic, the actual risk is much higher. Study after study has shown that most women who are heavy drinkers are also cigarette smokers. And as we shall see in Chapter 4, there is overwhelming evidence that smoking during pregnancy is a major contributor to the risk of giving birth to a small-for-dates baby. Thus, the woman who both drinks excessively and smokes regularly is increasing the chance of fetal growth retardation in two different ways. Each of these life-style habits can contribute independently to the slowed growth of the fetus, and to make matters more serious, the two risks add together. As a result, for the woman who both smokes and abuses alcohol, the probability of bearing a child whose growth is retarded in the womb is a whopping 400 percent greater than for the woman who neither smokes nor abuses alcohol.

Abnormalities of the Central Nervous System

The second major criterion for assigning the fetal alcohol syndrome label is a deficiency of the central nervous system, which includes the brain and spinal cord. Dysfunctions and abnormalities here take a variety of forms. Some symptoms can be seen within the first few days of life, while others may not show themselves until the child is ~al years of age. One of the symptoms seen in young ~ is an exaggerated tremulousness. It is important to emphasize "exaggerated." Virtually all babies have tremors, which look like shivering and usually involve the hands, feet, and possibly the jaw. In FAS babies, however, the tremors occur much more frequently, are more vigorous, and last for a longer period of time than in healthy newborns.

In parallel fashion, the babies diagnosed as exhibiting the fetal alcohol syndrome demonstrate frequent and an unusual amount of jitteriness and irritability. The abnormal increase in behavior such as tremors, jitters, and irritability is a sign that portions of the nervous system, including the brain, are not functioning in a normal way.

Another way in which the infant's exterior behavior can be examined in order to fathom the inner workings of the nervous system is by keeping track of sleep. Even at birth, a healthy newborn shows definite sleep-wake cycles and patterns of light and deep sleep. The regulation and organization of such patterns require a well-functioning nervous system. A group of researchers monitered three-day-old babies for a 24-hour period and found that the infants born to alcoholics showed much more disorganized sleep patterns and cyclicity than are usually seen. They were more restless than normal babies, and awake periods frequently interrupted their sleep. Although these findings were based on studying only a few babies, this work provides further evidence of a dysfunction in the organization and competence of the nervous systems of alcoholics' offspring.

Many, if not all, of the symptoms associated with the nervous system that are seen in these babies' first few days of life are also seen when adults stop heavy long-term alcohol drinking. Withdrawing adults go through a reaction marked by tremors, jitteriness, irritability, and sleep disturbances. At birth, the child of an alcoholic mother is suddenly cut off from the source of alcohol. It is not surprising, therefore, to see the baby display a pattern of withdrawal similar to that of an adult. The idea of a

newborn's undergoing alcohol withdrawal is entirely consistent with what has been shown to occur when the
mother has depended on other, "harder" drugs during
pregnancy. For example, infants born to narcotic users go
through several days of marked withdrawal on a much
more severe scale; symptoms include tremors, irritability,
vomiting, diarrhea, poor feeding, and shrill, high-pitched
crying.

Thus, to some degree, the abnormalities of the central
nervous system seen in the babies born to alcoholic mothers may be symptomatic of alcohol withdrawal. However,
most investigators believe that this early characteristic
behavior is indicative of more permanent dysfunction.
One would expect pure withdrawal effects to be relatively
temporary, lasting perhaps a week or so. But most of these
symptoms continue to manifest themselves in these children long after infancy. Apparently, alcohol withdrawal
makes an additional assault on the already compromised
nervous system of the baby who has been exposed to large
amounts of alcohol in the uterus.

As babies with the fetal alcohol syndrome get older,
they often show impairments or slowed development of
fine movements, such as the individual finger articulations
involved in picking and grasping objects, as well as a delay
in gross muscular movements, such as those used in
crawling, stepping and eye-hand coordination. There is
also a general tendency toward less-than-normal tone,
vigor, and tension in the muscles.

Signs of abnormalities in the central nervous system
continue as FAS babies grow. Their general behavior is
characterized by such traits as hyperactivity, difficulty in
paying attention, and nonspecific discoordinated movements. Together, these aspects of damage to the central
nervous system contribute to the most important consequence of alcoholism during pregnancy—a decrease in the
child's mental competence, ranging from borderline to
retarded intelligence. This effect is considered the most

serious of maternal drinking because reduced intellectual capabilities are the most debilitating, far-reaching, and tragic of all the features that make up the fetal alcohol syndrome. [1]

Various intelligence tests have been given to FAS children in hospitals and research facilities throughout the world, and the results have been disturbingly but strikingly similar. The first report, and the one that set the tone for those that followed, appeared in the scientific press just a year after the coining of the label and, in fact, was carried out by the University of Washington researchers who gave the syndrome its name. The children were part of an enormous prospective study involving 12 U.S. hospitals, 55,000 women and their offspring who had been observed for as long as seven years. Among the seven-year-old children of the alcoholics in the study, 44 percent scored at or below a level considered borderline retarded. Only 11 percent of a comparison group scored at or below this level. The evidence of lowered intelligence was not restricted to formal IQ tests. The offspring of alcoholics also performed consistently less well than the control group in tests of academic achievement, reading, arithmetic, and spelling.

In studies since 1974, some researchers have focused on assessing the intelligence of individuals who show FAS's physical features (growth retardation and specific facial characteristics). They have found that the intelligence scores are related to the severity or extent of the physical abnormalities contributing to the diagnosis of the fetal alcohol syndrome. For example, one study that examined 20 children of alcoholic mothers categorized the offspring, according to appearance, as having severe, moderately severe, moderate, mild, or very mild FAS physical features. After administering age-appropriate intelligence tests, the researchers looked at the relationship between the scores and the categories of physical abnormality. Among the five children with severe signs of the fetal alcohol syndrome, all had intelligence scores that ranked them as mentally deficient. Those who had been considered as showing moderately severe signs fared, on average, only slightly better; four of the five in this category scored in the mentally deficient range. Among the five considered to show moderate signs of FAS physical abnormalities, one had an intelligence score clearly in the mentally deficient range whereas the remaining four were borderline. Among the five remaining children, who displayed the least degree of physical abnormality, two tested in the mentally deficient range, one scored in the low-average category, and two were assessed as having average intelligence.

The irreversibility of the mental impairments following fetal exposure to alcohol is shown by the fact that five of the twenty children studied had been raised from birth in foster homes and certainly had had the benefit of a favorable home environment. (Some of the other children may have been raised in equally positive settings, but because the foster homes were carefully screened, one can be confident in making a judgment about them.) If the environment after birth were a critical factor in determining the presence or absence of mental handicaps among the offspring of the alcoholic mothers, one could reasonably expect somewhat higher intelligence scores among the fostered children. But the average ratings of the five fostered children did not differ from those of the others.

Follow-up studies gave more evidence that the prenatal consequences of alcohol exposure predominate over postnatal environmental factors. They also suggested the permanence of such effects. Seventeen of the children were retested one to four years after the original assessment. More than three-quarters of them had scores that were quite similar to those obtained on the initial test.

Although varying degrees of mental handicap are the most consistent as well as the most obvious sign of central-nervous-system dysfunction among FAS children, somewhat less debilitating abnormalities have also been found to be associated with maternal alcoholism. One investigation that illustrated this point used a procedure that was, in a sense, the reverse of the tactics described so far. Rather than examine children born to known alcoholics, the researchers chose to determine how many children referred to a clinic because of behavioral and learning difficulties in school had been exposed to heavy doses of alcohol during gestation. The results were startling.

During the one-year period while this study was underway, 15 of 87 children who came to the clinic had mothers who had a history of alcoholism during pregnancy. Those 15, representing 18 percent of the entire group, had a number of symptoms consistent with the fetal alcohol syndrome, including low weight at birth and low body weight, height, and head circumference at the time of referral. As well, all of them had some of the facial characteristics of the fetal alcohol syndrome, although all were in the normal range of intelligence. Not surprisingly, since the children had been referred to the clinic because of learning and behavioral problems at school, all had difficulties with attention and hyperactivity to the point of failure early in their educational experience. Unless in one-to-one or small group situations, they were unable to function, and their school records all contained descriptions such as "cannot sit still, easily distracted" or "behind ever since he entered school." The extreme nature of their difficulties was reflected by the fact that 13 of the 15 were referred to the clinic by the first grade.

These findings are noteworthy in their evidence of damage to the central nervous systems of the offspring of women who were alcoholics during pregnancy, even if the children have normal intelligence as measured in standardized tests. The form of the dysfunction is relatively subtle, taking on such aspects as learning and behavioral problems. Its appearance in conjunction with other symptoms of the fetal alcohol syndrome suggests that it may be at the lower end of the continuum of damage to the nervous system, becoming apparent only when the child encounters relatively stringent demands, such as those that occur in the classroom.

Facial Anomalies

Although growth retardation is possibly the easiest FAS symptom to measure and mental deficiences are the most dramatic, both can also be characteristic of a host of other conditions that have prenatal origins. Consequently, in designating a specific pattern of abnormalities as having been produced in the womb by alcohol, the syndrome's cluster of facial anomalies becomes an important, feature.

The facial anomalies that are part of FAS are not very dramatic, but they are striking enough for someone trained in recognizing physical abnormalities or someone who knows the specific aspects to look for. Two figures reproduced here show these aspects: one is a composite drawing of the facial features characteristic of FAS syndrome, while the other is a photograph of an eight-month-old baby diagnosed as having the syndrome.

Working from the top down, the first feature is the small head circumference, which is also an indicator of retarded growth. The region of the eyes often displays a number of anomalies. The most consistently reported is unusually small openings, which make the eyes look widely spaced. Many FAS children also have vertical folds of skin on the nasal side of the eyes, as well as drooping eyelids. The nose tends to be short and upturned (a "trumpet" nose), and the ridges running between the nose and mouth may be absent or indistinct. The upper lip tends to be thin and the chin small. Overall, the midface region is somewhat underdeveloped and flat.

Not all FAS children show all of these facial anomalies, but researchers have proposed that the label be reserved for individuals who have at least three clusters of them: a head circumference smaller than that of 97 percent of the "normal" population; small eye slits or poorly developed

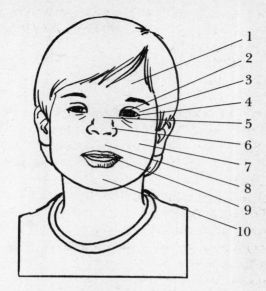

Facial Features Characteristic of the Fetal Alcohol Syndrome

Source: Adapted from Ann Pytkowicz Streissguth, Sharon Landesman-Dwyer, Joan C. Martin, and David W. Smith, "Teratogenic Effects of Alcohol in Humans and Laboratory Animals," *Science* 209 (reprint series, 18 July 1980): 355.

1 Small head circumference

2 Skin folds on nasal side of eyes

3 Drooping eyelids

4 Short eye openings

5 Low nasal bridge

6 Short nose

7 Flat midface

8 Indistinct ridges between nose and mouth

9 Thin upper lip

10 Small chin

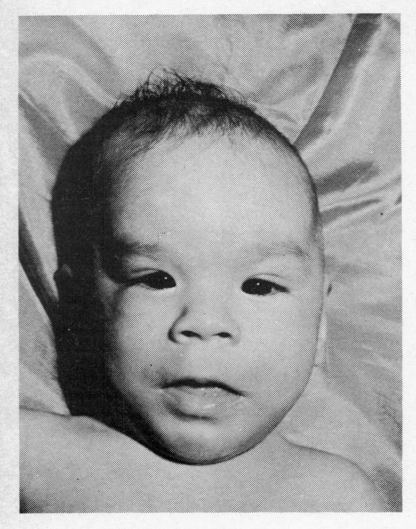

An Infant with the Fetal Alcohol Syndrome

Source: Reprinted with permission from Ann Pytkowicz Streiss-guth, Sharon Landesman-Dwyer, Joan C. Martin, and David W. Smith, "Teratogenic Effects of Alcohol in Humans and Laboratory Animals," *Science* 209 (reprint series 18 July 1980): 355.

ridges between the nose and mouth; and a thin upper lip or flat midface.

It is the presence of growth deficiences, central-nervous-system dysfunction, and a group of facial anoma-lies that defines the fetal alcohol syndrome. However, these children also have certain other anomalies with a greater-than-chance frequency. For example, heart defects occur in about 30 percent of the children diagnosed as having the syndrome, and minor problems with joints and genitals have been reported in several studies.

THE OCCURANCE OF THE FETAL ALCOHOL SYNDROME

How prevalent is the fetal alcohol syndrome among children born to alcoholic mothers? How common is the full-blown syndrome in the population at large? Concern about the frequency of the syndrome occurred, quite naturally, almost as soon as it was identified and labeled. The first, 1974 finding was a one-quarter frequency among the offspring of alcoholics. More recent clinical work, done in Sweden and Germany as well as the United States, agrees, reporting rates of 20 to 43 percent.

The question arises as to why the syndrome is not seen in *all* children of alcoholics. The answer is simply not known. It seems certain that a mother must be a heavy drinker throughout her pregnancy in order to give birth to a baby with fetal alcohol syndrome. This finding is completely consistent with the nature of the syndrome's anomalies. As we saw in Chapter 1, different parts and systems of the developing child are particularly vulnerable at different times during gestation. The facial abnormali-ties of the syndrome are most likely produced by high levels of alcohol concentration during the first trimester when the organs, limbs, and face are being formed. Since growth takes place primarily during the second and third trimester, this aspect of the syndrome is probably caused by heavy drinking during that period. Because much of the critical growth and development of connections in the nervous system occur late in pregnancy, the mental retardation and other behavioral and learning abnormalities may result from large amounts of alcohol being drunk during the third trimester.

Even through several researchers have found a greater likelihood of a FAS child among the most severe alcoholics (one estimate is a 43 percent rate) compared to women with milder alcoholism (an estimated rate of 20 percent), no one has discovered an upper level of consumption at which one can predict with certainty that the child will show all the symptoms associated with the fetal alcohol syndrome. For that matter, no upper level has been found beyond which even *some* alcohol effects always appear. Apparently, a host of other factors, including binge drinking habits, nutritional intake, the use of other drugs, and genetic makeup, enter into determining the risk factor.

Some researchers have said that the risk of the fetal alcohol syndrome may depend not so much on the exact amount of alcohol drunk but rather on the length of time the mother has been an alcoholic. Other published studies have reported that the likelihood of the syndrome is greater among the lower socioeconomic classes. Possibly, such women add the risk imposed by alcoholism to that of other adverse factors, such as poor nutrition, other drug use, and general poor health.

Does Male Drinking Play a Role?

Whether the father's drinking habits contribute to the fetal alcohol syndrome is a topic that has intrigued a number of researchers. Certainly, the notion that a father's heavy drinking can damage the offspring has a long history. Research in the last decade with rats and mice supports this contention; fetal deaths and growth retardation have been found among the offspring of matings between females with no access to alcohol and males fed a diet containing alcohol. In humans, the issue still remains to be examined in a carefully controlled fashion. It is known that alcohol affects some of the male hormones involved in reproduction, but whether such alterations have consequences for the offspring has not been established. A Boston study found that 30 percent of the heavy-drinking mothers it covered were associated with heavy-drinking males but gave no indication as to whether the children were more at risk when both parents abused alcohol.

How Many Children?

Determining the exact number of FAS children in the overall population is an impossible task, but by using studies in which large numbers of babies are examined for the symptoms comprising the syndrome, workers have estimated that the rate of occurrence is in the neighborhood of one or two per thousand. This estimate has been arrived at in separate studies in such diverse locations as France, Sweden, and the United States. In America, this rate of fetal alcohol syndrome works out to about four or five thousand births per year.

Presumably, the occurrence rate of just some of the FAS symptoms is much greater. One study carried out in Cleveland set the risk for individual alcohol-caused symptoms at an astounding 50 percent. This would translate into 80 to 100 thousand babies born in the United States each year who show some effects of maternal alcohol abuse. When one remembers that mental deficiency is one of the most frequent consequences, these figures become quite staggering. It is not surprising that one study concludes that "maternal abuse of alcohol during gestation... appears to be the most frequent known teratogenic cause of mental deficiency in the Western world."

WHEN SHOULD DRINKING BE REDUCED

The incidence of fetal alcohol effects is related to the amount of alcohol drunk during pregnancy. Therefore, a reduction in the risk of such adverse outcomes involves the reduction of alcohol use during gestation. However, that isn't the whole story. A history of heavy alcohol use also seems to play a role in increasing the risk factor.

How important is heavy drinking in producing risks for a yet-to-be-conceived baby? Although only a few studies have addressed this question, all of them have yielded results that point in the same direction.

The first study designed to look at this issue compared the birth weights of three groups of 50 babies. (The researchers chose this particular measurement because it is one of the most consistently affected features of fetal development as related to maternal drinking.) One group included infants born to women who had a history of alcoholism but reported total abstinence during pregnancy. Their alcoholism averaged seven years' duration before pregnancy, and they had stopped drinking an average of eight months before conceiving. The second group comprised infants born to women who continued to drink heavily during pregnancy. The last, a control group, included the newborn of nonalcoholic women who were essentially abstainers during pregnancy.

The birth weights of the babies showed a striking trend. Those infants born to the continuing alcoholics averaged about 18 ounces lighter than the babies born to the control subjects. The babies born to the abstinent alcoholics, although not as small as the infants of the continuing alcoholics, were still an average of 10 ounces smaller than the babies in the control group. These birth weight differences were not the result of such nonalcoholic factors as the mothers' ages or smoking habits.

Interestingly, the researchers could not relate the weights of the newborn of the abstinent alcoholics to the length of abstinence before conception. Studies using measures other than birth weight have, however, produced some evidence that the length of time a women has not abused alcohol prior to conception is related to the effects seen in her child. One study used scores on an intelligence test as a measurement of alcohol's effect. The children of abstinent alcoholics showed benefits if the mothers had stopped heavy drinking for at least a year before conception. The children of those who had abstained for less than a year were very similar to the children of the continuing alcoholics.

We do not know what biological factors cause the effects of prepregnancy alcoholism to persist when alcohol is not used during pregnancy. Some scientists have speculated, however, that alcoholic women may have so damaged their livers before conception that the food consumed during pregnancy is not used to a normal degree, with resulting nutritional problems for the developing fetus.

A German study used a slightly different approach to the issue. After examining the prepregnancy drinking history of mothers who had children showing at least some symptoms of the fetal alcohol syndrome, it ranked 108 children on the basis of the severity and number of alcohol effects and divided the mothers into three stages of alcoholism. In the mildest stage, the women drank excessively but were not recognized by society as alcoholics. The next stage was a loss of self-control, and the most severe stage was continuous drinking starting in the morning, with signs of biological and psychological damage. The investigators found that the degree of adverse consequences was related more to the degree of the mother's alcoholism than to the amount she drank during pregnancy or the number of years she had been drinking. The majority of children who had the full-blown fetal alcohol syndrome and showed the severest consequences of maternal alcohol abuse were born to mothers in the most advanced state of alcoholism.

Stopping Drinking during Pregnancy

In other words, the research suggests reasons for reducing or stopping drinking well before conception. Are there any measurable benefits if a heavy drinker stops drinking after she has discovered she is pregnant?

A team of medical personnel and social workers at the Boston City Hospital developed a strategy designed to assist pregnant alcoholics to reduce their intake markedly. They were told that heavy drinking might be harmful to the babies they were carrying and encouraged to attend counseling sessions scheduled to coincide with their routine prenatal appointments. In the counseling sessions, which were tailored to individual personal problems, the therapists also devoted considerable time to explaining how alcohol drunk by the mother crosses the placenta and reaches the fetus. They attempted to set up positive, supportive relationships, praising abstinence and avoiding direct criticism of drinking.

Among the 39 women who received counseling three or more times, 25 totally abstained or significantly reduced their drinking before the start of the third trimester. Their babies were compared to the 44 infants born to women who continued heavy drinking throughout pregnancy. In terms of growth, the differences between these two groups of babies were quite dramatic. Whether birth weight, length, or circumference was considered, moderation of drinking during pregnancy was associated with a greatly increased likelihood that the newborn would not be unusually small. The risk of fetal growth retardation was about five times higher for those babies born to women who did not reduce their drinking than for the infants of mothers who did.

These researchers encountered some difficulties in gathering objective measurements of abnormalities other than those related to growth. As a result, they reported data on physical anomalies and behavioral abnormalities, such as excess jitteriness, for only 15 babies whose mothers had reduced their drinking and 27 born to women who continued to drink heavily throughout pregnancy. Yet even with this small group of babies, the results were quite clear. Two-thirds of the babies born to women who had reduced their alcohol intake were diagnosed as normal, whereas only two of those born to the continuing alcoholics were given this clean bill of health. Also, more normal sleep patterns were observed among the babies who were not exposed to large amounts of alcohol during the third trimester.

German and Swiss studies have also noted marked benefits from reducing alcohol exposure late in pregnancy. They found that abnormalities were much less prevalent among the infants of alcoholics who reduced their drinking compared to the babies of women who continued to drink at alcoholic levels.

Clearly, the evidence suggests that the cessation of heavy drinking has definite advantages for the baby even if it occurs as late as the sixth month of pregnancy. The damage from heavy alcohol use that occurred early in pregnancy may not be reversible, but the risk to late fetal development, such as growth of the body and the nervous system, may be lowered by a significant reduction in alcohol intake during the last trimester. The evidence has led researchers in countries around the globe to conclude that the full fetal alcohol syndrome is seen only in the offspring of mothers who have drunk heavily throughout pregnancy.

CONCLUSION

The full fetal alcohol syndrome can be viewed as an anchor at one end of the spectrum of alcohol effects seen in babies who are born alive. Along the continuum toward normal, every subcombination of FAS anomalies can occur. As we have seen, there is no known amount of alcohol consumption above which the entire syndrome or some of its components always appear.

What about the mirror image of that issue? Is there a lower limit below which a pregnant woman's drinking will never produce any adverse effects in the baby she is carrying?

Before going on to that topic, it is worth pointing out that, as shown in the historical sketch at the beginning of this chapter, the sociopolitical climate has often affected the direction of science in the past. We are not immune to similar influences today. The current fashion is extreme sensitivity to environmental and life-style factors that may affect future generations. Yet it is important to avoid the temptation to exaggerate recent findings and the state of our knowledge. Only by presenting the facts as objectively as possible can we prevent a perpetuation of the unproductive historical cycle of acceptance, skepticism, rejection, and forgetfulness.

Alcohol: pregnancy and social drinking

Few researchers would take issue with the conclusion that very heavy drinking during pregnancy can have adverse consequences for the child. As we saw in Chapter 2, the evidence is too convincing and the potential effects too serious to have anything but a major impact upon the scientific community. Much more controversial, however, is the question of the possible consequences of more moderate levels of drinking.

For most people, the risk incurred by an alcoholic mother-to-be is someone else's problem. Any risks associated with more moderate drinking are more likely to strike home. Since more than 96 percent of women take at least an occasional drink, any effects on the fetus of moderate alcohol consumption have implications for a great number of mothers-to-be.

DEFINITIONS AND CATEGORIES OF DRINKING

One problem in any consideration of the use of alcohol is the definition of terms. Different people mean different things when they speak of "a moderate drinker" or "a heavy social drinker."

Most researchers believe that the categorization of drinkers should establish both the amount of alcohol consumed and the pattern of consumption. Many studies determine categories by asking a series of questions similar to those in the self-test reproduced here. Why don't you answer them and see how you might be labeled as a drinker?

WHAT KIND OF A DRINKER ARE YOU

Define one drink as a one bottle or can of regular beer, one glass (five ounces) of wine, or one highball or shot of "hard" liquor (one and a half ounces of any distilled alcohol). Answer the following questions, remembering to consider all three kinds of drinks.

1. On average, how often during the past year did you have a drink?

   a. More than once a day.
   b. Approximately once a day.
   c. Three to five times a week.
   d. About once or twice a week.
   e. Less than once a week but more than once a month.
   f. Less than once a month but more than once a year.
   g. Once a year or less.

2. On average, how much do you usually drink at one sitting?

   a. More than six drinks.
   b. Five to six drinks.
   c. Three to four drinks.
   d. One or two drinks.
   e. Less than one drink.

3. How often during the past year did you have five or six drinks at one sitting?

    a. nearly every time I drank.
    b. more than half the times I drank.
    c. sometimes.
    d. rarely.
    e. never.

Your answers to these questions reveal both your usual drinking habits and any bursts of heavy drinking that you indulge in. Using your answers, put yourself in one of the following categories.

Abstaining/infrequent drinker: Includes nondrinkers to those who drink less than once a month and never drink more than three drinks in one sitting.

Light/intermediate drinker: Includes those who drink at least once a month but less than once a week and never more than five drinks at one sitting to those who drink once or twice a week and rarely more than three or four drinks at one sitting.

Moderate drinker: Includes those who consume an average of three drinks a week to one drink a day and rarely more than three or four drinks at one sitting or those who drink once or twice a month and often have five or six drinks in one sitting.

Heavy drinker: Includes those who have an average of at least two drinks a day or those who average a drink a day and sometimes have five or six in one sitting.

Drinkers: Categories before and during Pregnancy

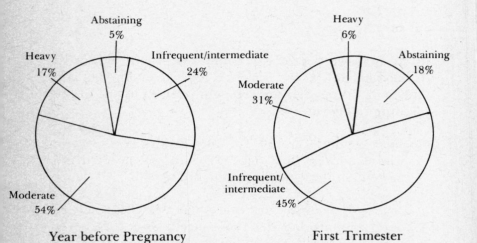

Year before Pregnancy

First Trimester

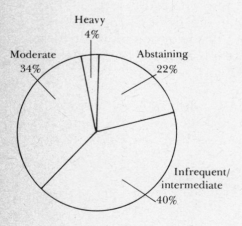

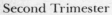

Second Trimester

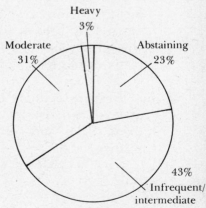

Third Trimester

Binge Drinking before and during Pregnancy

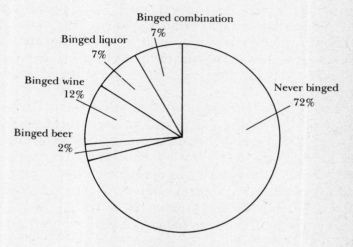

Binged combination
7%

Binged liquor
7%

Binged wine
12%

Binged beer
2%

Never binged
72%

Year before Pregnancy

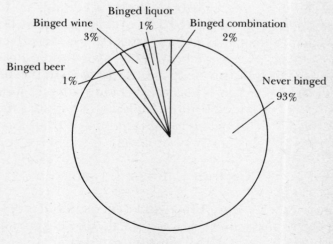

Binged wine
3%

Binged liquor
1%

Binged combination
2%

Binged beer
1%

Never binged
93%

During Pregnancy

The answers to such a combination of questions give a picture of two vital aspects of drinking behavior: the amount of alcohol drunk and the pattern of drinking, including both the individual's typical habits and any binge drinking. (As the phrase implies, binge drinking is having a large number of drinks over a short period of time, the kind of drinking that may occur at a party. Most researchers quantify a binge as five or more drinks within an hour or two). Using this information, researchers have developed criteria for the categories shown at the bottom of the self-quiz.

Two sets of graphs diagram the results of the responses of 700 women. The first shows the percentages who fell into each of the four drinking categories according to their habits in the year before they became pregnant and then during each trimester of pregnancy. The second set of graphs indicates the proportion of women who binge drank before and during pregnancy.

How do your drinking habits compare to those in the graphs?

In considering the definitions used, note that the "heavy drinker" category is open ended. A woman who falls at the lowest level of this category would, according to most people's norms, be considered a social drinker, albeit a heavy one. The problem in examining research reports occurs at the other end of this category. Since many studies use no upper cutoff, some of their findings on women they label "heavy drinkers" may reflect the drinking habits of women who drank considerably more than the minimum level of this category. This chapter's descriptions of studies point out those with this potential problem.

ALCOHOL AND THE FETUS

Like other forms of food and drink, alcohol is readily absorbed from the intestine into the bloodstream, but unlike carbohydrates and fats, it cannot be stored effectively in tissue. The body, therefore, has the task of disposing of virtually all the alcohol drunk, and it is the liver that has to do the work.

Since the placenta does not act as a barrier to alcohol's reaching the fetus, it is not surprising that the concentration of alcohol in an unborn baby's blood is quite similar to the concentration in the mother's. If the pregnant woman drinks enough to get drunk, her baby is also exposed to that level of alcohol.

Here arises the potential problem of binge drinking by an otherwise moderate mother-to-be. The sudden influx of alcohol from such a drinking bout may well affect whatever development the unborn baby is undergoing at the time. Importantly, the adult is capable of eliminating alcohol from her body at a considerably faster rate than the fetus. So once alcohol crosses the placenta, it remains in the baby's system for a longer time than a similar amount would remain in the mother's. Presumably, the longer the alcohol stays in the body, the greater its potential for adverse effects.

How long alcohol stays in the system depends in part on the functioning of the liver, which for the fetus, depends on the age. A third-trimester fetus can break down alcohol, but because its liver is not fully mature, it gets rid of the drug at less than half the adult rate. In the first or second trimester, the elimination rate is even slower because the young fetus is dependent upon the mother to get rid of alcohol. Once alcohol crosses the placenta, it circulates through the baby's system and is removed only when it recrosses, via the umbilical arteries, to the mother and is processed by her liver. Relative to an adult's system of alcohol disposal, this process is lengthy indeed.

A Treatment That Provided Clues

A major impetus for studying the consequences of alcohol metabolism in pregnancy arose in a somewhat strange fashion in the mid-1960s. Because of the high incidence of mortality, sickness, and abnormalities in infants born prematurely, physicians have long been searching for a pharmacological method of stopping labor if it begins before the fetus is suitably mature. Consequently, a 1967 report aroused considerable interest with its description of prevention of early labor by administering alcohol intravenously to the mother. Although this procedure is rarely used today because of adverse side effects, it was found effective for about two-thirds of all patients treated; in about one-third of these cases, delivery was delayed for at least four weeks.

The amount of alcohol the mother received in this treatment was considerable—enough to get her inebriated. In some of the cases in which it did not successfully stop labor, infants were born with considerable amounts of alcohol in the blood and even their breath smelled of alcohol. The speed with which this substance passed from mother to baby was dramatically seen in a report that described alcohol being injected two minutes before delivery and found in the infant immediately after the birth.

Researchers are particularly interested in this medical use of alcohol because any effects seen in the newborn under controlled conditions that specify the quantity of maternal alcohol intake can serve as a barometer of what may happen if the fetus is briefly exposed to large amounts of alcohol. In other words, the injection of alcohol to curtail early labor can be used as a model of binge drinking during pregnancy.

Some doctors found that the alcohol given to arrest labor tended to inhibit the breathing of the newborn. Is there a parallel effect on the fetus? In spite of the absence of air to breathe in the uterus, the fetus begins to exhibit rhythmic movements of the wall of the chest and diaphragm during the second trimester. Amniotic fluid moves in and out of the passages of the respiratory tract in response to these fetal breathing movements, which are thought to be forerunners of breathing air after birth.

The fetal breathing movements increase in rate as birth approaches; chest expansion and relaxation occur approximately thirty times per minute. These movements are quite complex, involving a large number of muscles that move in a coordinated fashion, following a definite sequence. Since such a reflex must be directed by portions of the brain, these breathing movements, which can be monitored by ultrasound, can serve as a reflection of the development of components of the central nervous system.

In one study, women in their last month of pregnancy who reported that they normally drank one to three cocktails per week were given one ounce of vodka mixed with ginger ale. Within 30 minutes, monitoring revealed a marked suppression of the fetal respiratory movements, and it lasted as much as an hour. This result shows that when even a limited amount of alcohol is consumed, it can pass rapidly from mother to baby, and it apparently can depress at least certain activities of the fetal nervous system.

STUDIES OF STILLBIRTHS AND MISCARRIAGES

A number of studies have directly addressed various aspects of the question of whether drinking at nonalcoholic levels affects the fetus. Some, have focused on relatively subtle phenomena, while others have looked at life-threatening situations.

The 1976 French Study

In 1976, a group of French scientists collected information on more than 9,000 pregnancies, interviewing the women during the first trimester and obtaining reports on the outcomes of the pregnancies. The data collected included the alcohol consumption of each mother-to-be.

The researchers divided the subjects into categories ranging from those who abstained to those who drank more than two ounces of absolute alcohol (that is, more than the equivalent of three cocktails) per day during the pregnancy.

Among those women who reported abstaining during pregnancy, the stillbirth rate was 9.5 per thousand. Among the women in the heaviest drinking category, it was 37.4 per thousand. That works out to an increase of approximately 400 percent in risk! Among the women who averaged 1.5 to 2.0 ounces of absolute alcohol (two to three cocktails) a day, the risk was 22.4 per thousand—approximately midway between the rate for the group of heaviest drinkers and for the nondrinkers.

In 1980, the French workers reported data from two newer studies. The trend of an increase in stillbirths among women who drank more than 1.5 ounces of absolute alcohol per day was still evident, but it was not as clear as in the earlier study. Possibly contributing to this lessening of significance were the smaller number of women participating in the later project (about a third of the earlier sample size) and the fact that the overall stillbirth rate was down by about 40 percent, making it more difficult to detect alcohol's effects.

The 1976 French study was important not only because of its size but also because it considered the type of alcohol consumed. The women who drank were divided into three groups: those who consumed wine only, those who drank beer only, and those who consumed both. (Cider was included in the beer category. Beer, wine, and cider were thought to account for nearly all of the alcohol consumed by French women). When one compares the stillbirth rate of the heavier drinkers in each of the three beverage categories, beer appears to have a special role. The heavy beer and beer-plus-wine drinkers had an increased risk for stillbirths that was three to four times greater than the light drinkers, whereas those women who drank only wine did not increase their risk of stillbirth at all. Whether these findings reflect some special property of the different types of beverages or whether there are some nonalcoholic risk factors for stillbirths that are more common among beer drinkers than among wine drinkers remains to be determined. Certainly the issue needs further investigation.

A Large American Study

In an American study, more than 32,000 women completed a questionnaire on alcohol use in pregnancy. Approximately half of the women reported that they did not drink during the pregnancy, and about 3 percent had one or more drinks a day.

Among the women who drank on a regular, daily basis, there was a clear increase in the rate of spontaneous abortions, particularly in the second trimester. The risk increased with the amount drunk. For those who had one or two drinks a day, the risk was almost twice as great as for nondrinkers, while the women who averaged more than three drinks a day were three and a half times more likely than nondrinkers to have a spontaneous abortion.

The very large number of subjects in this study made it possible for the researchers to consider subgroups of women who were at risk for miscarriages for reasons other than alcohol. For example, women who were older and did not drink were compared to women of similar age who did consume alcohol. Other factors that were considered in this manner included smoking, race (blacks have a relatively high miscarriage rate), and previous history of spontaneous abortions. In all the subgroups, the women who drank more than one drink a day had a consistently higher risk for second-trimester miscarriages.

This study found no consistent increased rate of spontaneous abortions among the women who drank less than once a day. However, this finding may be somewhat misleading because of the way the drinking was categorized. The questionnaire given the women asked: "During the first three months of this pregnancy ... did you take any alcoholic beverages? If yes, did you average six or more drinks a day, three to five, one to two, or less than one drink daily?" Notice that this lumps together all women who drank anything from the tiniest amount up to six drinks a week. It is possible that women who drank at the upper end of this scale may have run a higher risk than the very light drinkers, but this could not be determined because they were all considered together. For example, any effect from six drinks a week might have been counterbalanced by an absence of effects from one drink a week and so not reflected in the group average. Thus, the finding that, as a group, the women who drank less than one drink did not differ from the nondrinkers does not automatically mean that the "safe" level of alcohol consumption with respect to spontaneous abortions is just under a drink a day.

A New York Study of Spontaneous Abortion

A group of New York investigators did attempt to see if the risk for miscarriages is higher among women who drink at levels well under once a day. This study examined the alcohol habits of 616 women who had aborted spontaneously. They were interviewed in hospitals after being admitted because of miscarriage; a comparison group was comprised of age-matched women in postnatal outpatient clinics who had given birth in the same hospitals. The investigators reported an increased risk of spontaneous abortions in women who were categorized as drinking two to six times a week where the average drink per occasion was a minimum of one ounce of absolute alcohol (roughly, two bottles of beer, two mixed drinks, or two four-ounce glasses of wine). Twice as many of the women who miscarried reported drinking at this level as did those women who had successful births. This ratio held when other, nonalcohol risk factors were taken into consideration.

Several things should be noted about this study. First, it made no breakdown of the frequency of drinking within the two-to-six-times-a-week group, so one cannot conclude that the low end of this category carries the same risk as the upper end. Second, the researchers found that the major difference between the women who miscarried and those who did not was how often they drank—not how much they drank at each sitting. Whether this finding would hold true for the ingestion of larger amounts of alcohol is another issue. Finally, this study, like the French one, looked at different types of alcoholic beverages—in this case, beer, wine, and spirits. Taking into account the level of absolute alcohol in each, the three did not differ from one another in their contribution to the risk of spontaneous abortion. This part of the report appears to be at odds with the French investigation, which found beer to be a greater contributing factor to stillbirths than wine. Whether the inconsistency in the two studies reflects the different mechanisms underlying abortions and stillbirths, differences in European and American alcohol, or some other factor must await further research.

Fetal Loss: Conclusions

On the basis of most of the data, one can conclude that drinking more than three ounces of absolute alcohol per week is associated with a measurable increase in fetal loss. As the alcohol consumption increases, so does the risk. The lower limit has not been established and is unlikely ever to be so. Genetic differences and nonalcoholic risk factors make it virtually impossible for researchers to come up with a "safe" amount with universal applicability.

INVESTIGATIONS OF COMPLICATIONS OF PREGNANCY AND BIRTH WEIGHT

Other complications associated with nonalcoholic levels of drinking may not lead to the death of the unborn baby but are still of great concern because of their consequences for the child.

Abruptio Placenta

Because the placenta is such a complex organ that must perform so many functions vital to fetal life, growth, and development and because it is so exposed to alcohol consumed by the mother, many researchers think it a key target for any adverse effects that might be caused by drinking. One problem they have looked at is abruptio placenta, the premature separation of some of the placenta from the wall of the uterus. This is a very serious condition because it interrupts the oxygen supply to the fetus. If only a small area of the placenta separates and the fetus can be delivered quickly, the outcome may be a live, healthy baby. On the other hand, if too much of the placenta separates, the baby cannot survive.

The French study already described found a marked increase in the risk of abruptio placenta among the women who drank more than 1.5 ounces of absolute alcohol a day. In fact, according to the investigators, severe abruptio was the major cause of stillbirths that appeared to be associated with alcohol.

It is important to note that cigarettes have also been found to increase the risk of this condition. Therefore, the woman who both smokes and drinks heavily during pregnancy is running a particularly high risk of this serious complication.

Reduced Birth Weight

Since reduced birth weight has been a consistent finding among infants born to alcoholics, it is not surprising that this measure of intrauterine growth is one of the primary targets for determining whether more moderate levels of drinking can influence fetal development. The 1976 French study noted that for the infants of women who reported abstaining during pregnancy, the average birth weight was 7.30 pounds. Women who drank two to three drinks a day had infants weighing an average of 7.20 pounds. Women in the heaviest drinking category, with a daily average consumption of at least three drinks a day (notice the open upper end), had the smallest babies, with an average weight of 7.07 pounds. The difference in birth weight between the children borne by the heavy social drinkers and by the abstainers was consistent but not large—only four ounces.

Most, although not all, subsequent studies have confirmed the French conclusion that drinking at nonalcoholic levels during pregnancy is associated with a small reduction in birth weight. For example, the first American study designed to gather information about birth weight and social drinking was reported in 1977. The subjects were 263 middle-class, primarily white women in the Seattle area who were interviewed in their fifth and eighth month of pregnancy. After taking into account the smoking habits of the mother, the sex of the child, the mother's age and height, and other factors that play a role in determining weight, the researchers concluded that drinking an average of two drinks per day late in pregnancy was associated with a 5.5-ounce decrease in birth weight, a finding slightly more pronounced than that of the earlier French study.

Three reports have cropped up in which the authors have failed to find a relationship between drinking during pregnancy and the size of the newborn baby. Interestingly, two of these studies simply divided pregnant women into two large categories: those who reported that they were nondrinkers and those who reported drinking at any level. Given reports that heavy social drinking, if it affects the weight of the newborn, does so only slightly, it is not surprising that this broad categorization, which put light and moderate drinkers in the same group as heavy drinkers, did not reveal any detectable relationship between alcohol and birth weight.

In the third study that reported no correlation between nonalcoholic levels of drinking and fetal growth, the
absence of a relationship may well be because the group
included such a small number of women who drank at
levels that other researchers have associated with low birth
weight. Only nine women in this study drank 1.5 drinks or
more per day in the first trimester, and by the third
trimester the number was reduced to four. Given this
limited number of subjects, it is not surprising that the
slight effect of heavy social drinking was not picked up. A
relatively large number of observations have to be made to
confirm the presence of any phenomenon that is small in
nature.

STUDIES OF NEWBORNS' BEHAVIOR

If social drinking can slow the growth of the fetus even
slightly, it may also affect more subtle aspects of development, ones that are not as easy to assess. Some researchers
have attempted to determine whether it has measurable
effects on the behavior of babies during the first few days
of life.

The Seattle Study

Since most of the data in this area has come from the
Seattle study that began in late 1974 and is still going on,
it is worth looking at its procedures in a little detail.

All pregnant women receiving prenatal care during
1974 and 1975 in two hospitals in Seattle were asked to
participate in the study. More than 1,500 women agreed to
a 30-minute interview conducted in the fifth month of
pregnancy. Among the many questions asked were some
about their drinking and smoking habits before and
during pregnancy. Alcohol ingestion was recorded by both
the amount drunk and the pattern of drinking. Approximately 500 of the women were followed up after they gave
birth. Of these, 250 were women who were categorized as

heavy drinkers (two or more drinks a day or occasional binges); the remaining 250 were rare or infrequent drinkers who served as a comparison or control group.

The babies of these 500 women were examined at a variety of ages. Medical records of Apgar test results were used to chart them immediately after birth. Among the infants born to heavy social drinkers, the risk for an Apgar score of three or less (out of a possible ten) at one minute after birth was found to be 7 percent. For the infants of the remaining women, the risk was only 3 percent. Although not dramatic, this finding indicates that heavy social drinking during pregnancy involves an increased risk of difficulties for the offspring immediately after birth.

Further studies by the Seattle researchers lead to the conclusion that effects associated with heavy social drinking can be found beyond the first moments of life in the outside world. The Brazelton Neonatal Behavioral Scale was administered to the babies at 8 to 36 hours of age to assess the way in which they interacted with their new environment. Two general findings emerged. First, compared to the babies of abstainers or light drinkers, the babies of heavy drinkers took longer before they habituated to redundant stimuli. This slower rate is suggestive because fairly rapid habituation in appropriate situations is a useful adaptive ability thought to be an early measure of the functioning of the nervous system. Second, the babies of the heavy drinkers differed from those of the light drinkers in general level of behavior. The former were characterized as having low arousal levels; they seldom became very upset or excited, and when they did cry, they were easy to console and frequently quieted themselves. During the examination period, they also tended to alternate between awake and drowsy states rather than between awake and crying states.

The Implications of the Behavioral Studies

The logical question here is so what? What does it

matter that heavy social drinking during pregnancy may increase the chances of having a baby who is relatively passive in nature and who does not habituate as efficiently as others to repetitive stimuli?

The question can be tackled at several levels. At one level—a speculative one—it can be argued that low arousal may have a negative effect on the way the infant and mother relate to each other. There is evidence that the behavior of the newborn, particularly the way he or she reacts and interacts with the mother, is very important to bonding, that rapid process which creates a unique affectionate relationship between mother and baby shortly after birth. Infants whose behavior reveals low arousal may not elicit the same qualitative or quantitative reactions from their mothers as newborns who respond to the environment (including their mothers) with a wide range of emotions.

The reduced tendency to habituate with its concomitant diminished ability to select out stimuli to which attention ought to be paid may affect the newborn's ability to learn from the environment. Thus, an altered habituation rate in the day-old baby may have consequences for later development. These hypotheses are, of course, speculative and remain to be investigated in a rigorous fashion.

A second level is possible in answering the inquiry of so what. The subtle signs seen in the offspring of heavy social drinkers indicate that exposure of the fetus to non-alcoholic levels of alcohol increases the risk of an atypical newborn. One may wonder whether there are long-term effects, but that is not the only issue. One must also consider the newborn infant—if he or she is affected by the mother's alcohol consumption, *that* is a matter of concern in itself. According to this line of thinking, the newborn is an end product, not merely a preliminary step for some future stage of development. Thus, even if the effects disappear and have no measurable repercussions when the child is one year old, five years old, or whatever, the fact that they were present at all makes the findings important.

At a third, related level, the answer is that the behavior exhibited in the Brazelton examination may represent only *some* of the subtle consequences of social drinking during pregnancy. Other types of testing may reveal other effects.

Some More Seattle Studies

This tip-of-the-iceberg hypothesis gains support from other studies carried out by the Seattle investigators. They have looked at such things as general behavior, suckling, and learning ability in babies two days of age or less. In each study, the finding was the same: drinking at heavy but nonalcoholic levels during pregnancy was associated with an increased risk for an atypical newborn.

In one of these studies, babies 8 to 32 hours of age were placed in a quiet room in the hospital nursery after their early morning feeding. An observer closely monitored each infant's behavior for one and a half to two hours, noting all forms of external stimulation. Use of a specially developed electronic digital keyboard permitted a coded record to be kept of which of the baby's senses was being stimulated, whether the nurses were talking, and so on. The activities of the baby, including seven different types of eye movements (closed, squint, bright, and so on), eight types of vocalization and facial expressions, head movements, and limb activities were also encoded by pressing various numbers on the keyboard. The data were recorded on a cassette tape, which fed into a computer. The elaborate equipment permitted quick and accurate descriptions of 45 different types of naturally occurring behavior to determine whether the babies of heavy social drinkers were different than the offspring of infrequent drinkers. For several kinds of behavior, the answer appeared to be yes. The infants who had been exposed prenatally to relatively high doses of alcohol were more likely than their counterparts to display increased body tremors, decreased vigorous body activity, increased time in a nonalert awake state, and increased hand-to-mouth activity. Intriguingly, this behavior is similar to that observed in babies diagnosed as having the fetal alcohol syndrome and in babies undergoing narcotic withdrawal.

On the other hand, babies born to narcotics addicts and alcoholics are usually irritable and fussy, but the offspring of the heavy social drinkers were not. Why this was so remains a mystery at this time.

The established relationship between certain kinds of behavior in newborns and narcotics use or alcoholism during pregnancy was one of the major reasons for examining sucking behavior in the offspring of the social drinkers. Infants born to addicts and alcoholics have frequently been found to have a weaker suck than most other newborns. This decreased vigor in nursing is important partly because it is assumed to be one more subtle behavioral sign of central-nervous-system dysfunction and partly in its own right. Babies with a weaker suck often require longer and more frequent feedings and are more likely to fail to thrive since sucking pressure is directly related to milk intake. Because the weaker suck had been observed among the newborn of alcoholics, the Seattle group of researchers wondered whether a similar but presumably less-pronounced effect would be seen in the offspring of the heavy social drinkers. They used an apparatus consisting of an artificial nipple attached to a pressure-sensing device that could monitor the strength and frequency of sucking. The average pressure exerted on the nipple was indeed less among the babies born to the heavy social drinkers than among the other infants.

Another Seattle experiment made use of the fact that the baby can suck at birth to examine how newborns react to experience—a form of learning. The babies were given a nipple that did not provide them with any form of liquid. If they sucked ten times within a 30-second period, they were rewarded with a sip of glucose water. Then, after 20 such sequences, they no longer received the sweetened water. Thus, the experiment examined both the learning of the presence of a reward as well as how quickly the baby realized that he or she was no longer getting any reward, even after working for it. The researchers found that slower learning was generally associated with the infants of mothers who both drank and smoked during pregnancy. Neither social drinking nor a nicotine habit alone was related to slower-learning newborns.

Whether measures of learning during the first few days of life are in any way predictive of later learning is not known. However, the point is that the baby born to a heavy social drinker has an increased probability of being, during the first few days of life, different in a number of ways from infants born to abstainers or light drinkers.

STUDIES OF PHYSICAL ANOMALIES

One of the three criteria for labeling babies as having the fetal alcohol syndrome is the presence of minor physical anomalies. Is the child of a social drinker more likely than the child of a nondrinker to show such effects? Quite naturally, a number of researchers have asked this question. The final verdict is not in. Several studies, some of them large, have failed to find any association between social drinking and anomalies of the type seen in FAS infants, but other investigations have found such a link.

One study merits particular attention because it is widely cited as indicating that the risk for anomalies starts to increase with as few as one or two drinks per day. A total of 163 babies were examined for physical abnormalities. Approximately half the mothers reported drinking at least one and a half drinks per day or having had five or more drinks on at least one occasion during the pregnancy. The remaining women were abstainers or very light drinkers.

Eleven of the 163 babies showed some of the abnormalities associated with the fetal alcohol syndrome. Who were these eleven babies? Six were born to women who drank one and a half to three drinks per day and three were born to women who drank four or more drinks a day. What about the other two? Surprisingly, they were born to women who reported themselves as abstainers or very light drinkers. It is not known what factors caused these women to have infants with anomalies consistent with those seen in babies labeled as FAS infants. Possibly, it may reflect inaccurate reporting of alcohol habits or some nonalcohol influence.

What the data suggest is a relationship between the quantity drunk and the likelihood of finding an alcohol-related effect—in other words, a dose-response curve. The risk of the baby's showing signs of an alcohol-related physical anomaly goes up as the average daily consumption by the mother-to-be increases. Our understanding of this dose-response relationship is crude at this time as it is based on relatively few subjects. Clearly, the risk varies from one person to the next depending on a host of other factors. All the same, we have begun to establish a link between the amount drunk and the risk of certain aspects of the fetal alcohol syndrome. The work suggests that consumption of less than one drink a day results in a relatively low risk for the types of physical abnormalities associated with the fetal alcohol syndrome; consumption of about one and a half to three drinks per day increases the risk to about 11 percent; consumption at what many workers consider moderate levels ups the risk level to about 20 percent; and, as described in the previous chapter, severe alcoholism increases the risk to 40 percent or more.

These risk levels are relatively similar to those found in another research program set up at the Boston City Hospital, where 322 women registering for prenatal care were interviewed to determine their alcohol intake, then divided into heavy, moderate, and rare drinkers. When they gave birth, the babies were examined in the newborn nursery by doctors who did not know the drinking history of the mothers (to prevent bias in one direction or the other). Minor malformations were found in 5 percent of the offspring of the rare drinkers, 12 percent of the offspring of the moderate drinkers, and 17 percent of the offspring of the heavy drinkers.

Binge drinking may play an important role in the presence or absence of anomalies. As described in Chapter 1, we have quite complete knowledge of what develops at what stage in the growth of the embryo and fetus. Thus, we are on sound ground in hypothesizing that in order for alcohol to induce physical anomalies, it must be present in fairly high concentrations during the critical time in the first trimester when organ and facial development is taking place. This notion lessens the importance of average weekly consumption, particularly for social drinkers, and increases the importance of peak concentrations of alcohol in the mother's system—the kind that would occur during occasional binging. Unfortunately, it is early in pregnancy that the embryo is most susceptible to structural aberrations, and it is at this time, when pregnancy may not be recognized, that the mother-to-be is most likely to indulge in a binge.

STUDIES OF LATER DEVELOPMENT

The next step in determining alcohol-related risks is to look at the development of babies as they get older. Are there signs indicating that prenatal exposure to alcohol at social-drinking levels has any long-term, measurable influence on physical and mental development? The answer is maybe. Because the topic of social drinking and pregnancy is such a recent area of concern, very few research centers have reported data on any children of more than a few days old. What follows is essentially the total of our current knowledge. Its very brevity suggests how much remains to be ascertained, but at least the first steps have been taken. The currency of the information is highlighted by the fact that all of the available data have been published since 1980.

The West German Study

From Dusseldorf, West Germany comes a report based on almost 7,000 births between 1965 and 1972. Women were registered in this study during their first trimester and asked at that time about their use of alcohol. Unfortunately, the questions were phrased in such an imprecise and subjective manner that the results are very difficult to interpret. The women were asked which category they felt best described themselves: did they drink "not at all or occasionally," "a little every day," or "several times a day"? Since only 15 of the women placed themselves the heaviest drinking category, the researchers decided they had to base their report on the many more numerous women who reported drinking "a little every day." Their offspring were compared to the children of women who categorized themselves as abstainers or occasional drinkers. In all the aspects the German researchers looked at—growth, motor capabilities, general behavior, age at developmental milestones—they observed no differences between the children of the drinking and of the nondrinking mothers. The absence of any effect of alcohol in this work is difficult to interpret. It may be the real state of affairs. On the other hand, the study's lack of precision in categorizing maternal alcohol intake makes it unlikely that the workers could have picked up any but the most striking consequences.

The Seattle Study of Eight-Month-Olds

Two studies from the Seattle group of researchers tend to confirm this hypothesis. Both involved follow-up of some of the babies originally tested extensively during their first few days of life, as described earlier in this chapter. Results have been reported for children tested at eight months and at four years of age.

The development of the babies was assessed by a

widely used standardized procedure. A trained observer closely scrutinizes the infant in a variety of clearly specified situations using specific "toys" to elicit responses. The 30-minute test is divided into complementary parts. One examines the baby's ability to perceive and react to different sounds and sights, the beginnings of memory, and early vocalization; collectively, the results are considered to assess mental development. A second grouping of tests are thought to measure motor development; they look at control of the body, coordination of the large muscles, and finer manipulatory abilities of the hands and fingers. The purpose of both the mental and the motor tests is to compare the individual infant's development to what has been seen in a large number of previously tested babies. It is important to note, however, that the tests are not considered useful indictors of how the child will do in the future. Except in cases of extreme abnormality, infant behavioral tests have little predictive value. Their value lies in determining the current state of affairs, not in foretelling whether the baby will be a university graduate or a kindergarten dropout.

The Seattle researchers got similar results on the mental and the motor tests. Drinking during pregnancy was associated with subtle but consistently lower scores on both scales, and this effect did not correlate with nonalcohol factors, such as smoking, other drugs, educational level of the mother, or any obvious factor in the environment between birth and the time of testing. Because the researchers quantified the amounts of alcohol drunk by the women in the study, they were able to compare the babies of the abstainers and rare drinkers to the infants of women who drank two to four drinks a day and of those who drank more than four drinks daily. From the results, it appears that the minimum level of alcohol consumption that may affect the child's development is somewhere between three and four drinks a day.

The Seattle Study of Four-Year-Olds

As noted in Chapter 2, researchers have frequently found poor attention spans and fidgetiness in the children of alcoholics, even in those who do not show signs of mental retardation. Therefore, the Seattle researchers looked for similar behavioral problems in the four-year-old offspring of a number of women participating in the study. Combining the mother's own rating of her child's temperament with observations by trained personnel of the child at home during a meal, at play, and while being read a story by the mother, the researchers recorded the behavior of 128 children. Included in this group were 67 born to women who had drunk up to four drinks per day during pregnancy with an overall average of alcohol consumption of approximately one drink a day. These children were compared to the children of abstainers or rare drinkers. The researchers found that the offspring of the social drinkers tended to be more fidgety, less attentive, and less obedient than the other children. The differences were small and, at this time, can only be viewed as suggestive. Furthermore, whether the slight differences seen in the four-year-olds will remain or alter as they enter school is a question that cannot be answered for a year or two.

Several things in this study merit highlighting, however. The first is the parallel between the observed behavior of the children of the social drinkers and the children of alcoholics. Certainly, the effect is less, but the general behavior appears to be on the same continuum. Second, the home environments of children of the social drinkers and the nondrinkers did not differ in terms of stimulation available from books, toys, and so on. In fact, as measured by observers using specific criteria, most homes in the study provided an enriched environment. Third, the amount of alcohol consumed by these social drinkers was low. Couple this with the fact that the women in all the Seattle social-drinking studies were generally a low-risk population, and the results become more striking. These women were mostly middle class, received prenatal care, were well nourished, and did not use other drugs. Whether the levels of alcohol they reported drinking would show a more pronounced effect on mothers-to-be who are at risk for reasons not related to alcohol is a possibility that must be considered.

CONCLUSION

We have now come to the end of what is known about drinking in pregnancy at nonalcoholic levels. Clearly our knowledge in this area is not complete, but many studies provide at least preliminary evidence that the risks of adverse effects begin to increase at alcohol-consumption levels well below those of alcoholism or alcohol abuse. The influence of nonalcoholic levels of drinking during pregnancy can be summarized as likely affecting: (1) the risk level of spontaneous abortion and stillbirths; (2) the degree of fetal growth; (3) the occurence of physical anomalies; and (4) a variety of behavior in newborns, babies, and young children.

The minimum level of drinking that may affect the unborn child is still a controversial subject. It probably will remain so for some time as researchers attempt to understand and clarify dose levels, binge-drinking effects, timing, and individual differences. In spite of these unknown factors, this chapter can end with a fairly definite statement. No evidence indicates that total abstinence from alcohol is necessary for a healthy, pregnant woman. However, there are ample warning signals that what might be considered moderate social drinking is not enough moderation when a woman is pregnant.

4   Caffeine

Although caffeine does not have a history nearly as long as alcohol's, it has rapidly evolved into the world's most popular drug. Legend has it that caffeine's stimulative property was first observed in animals in the 15th century. Goatherds noted that their animals were restless and did not sleep at night after grazing on wild coffee beans. An astute holy man in Arabia realized that a drink made from these beans would help the devout to keep awake during the long nights of prayer at the mosque. This beverage was called *qahweh*, which translates from Arabic as that which stimulates or suppresses the appetite for food; the term is the origin of the words coffee and caffeine.

By the middle of the 15th century, coffee was a popular beverage in Arabia, and it spread quickly to Turkey, then to North African regions, and finally to Europe and North and South America. When first introduced to the Western world, coffee was thought of as an intoxicating beverage that was dangerous to health. How things have changed! Today coffee is a staple in more than 90 percent of North American households—the annual consumption of green coffee beans in the United States is more than two billion pounds.

SOURCES OF CAFFEINE

The amount of caffeine in a cup of coffee can vary enormously, ranging from 29 to 333 milligrams per cup. The type of bean used is one factor contributing to this variation. For example, beans grown in South and Central America contain about half as much caffeine as those grown in Africa. Another source of variation is the method of preparation, as well as the brand. For example, instant coffee ranges from 29 to 177 milligrams per cup with an average of about 66, percolated coffee averages 74 milligrams, and drip coffee 112. Decaffeinated coffee usually contains about 3 milligrams per cup.

Coffee accounts for about 75 percent of all the caffeine consumed in North America. The next most popular source is tea. North American instant tea averages about half as much caffeine as coffee, but in England, where the beverage is taken much stronger, the caffeine per cup is similar to that in a cup of coffee.

Cola drinks rank third, with half their caffeine coming from the kola nut used to flavor them and half added during manufacture. Relatively small amounts of caffeine also enter the diet via cacao beans, which are the major ingredient of chocolate, and in over-the-counter medicines, such as cold tablets, allergy and headache-relief pills, and "stay-awake" tablets.

The table in this chapter lists the amounts of caffeine in some common substances. The average consumption of caffeine in North America by men, women, and children is about 200 milligrams daily. (About half that amount taken at one time is enough to produce significant effects in most people.) Many individuals take in much larger amounts. One study found that about 25 percent of Americans ingest 500 to 600 milligrams per day, and 10 percent may take more than 800.

COMMON SOURCES OF CAFFEIN

	Average amount
Instant coffee	66 mg/cup
Percolated coffee	74 mg/cup
Drip coffee	112 mg/cup
Decaffeinated coffee	3 mg/cup
Tea	30 mg/cup
Cola	50 mg/cup
Cocoa	35 mg/cup
Chocolate bar	25 mg
Cold tablet	23 mg
Allergy-relief tablet	16 mg
Headache-relief tablet	64 mg
"Stay-awake" tablet	150 mg

Caffeine is usually thought of as a substance that is almost exclusively in the domain of adults. However, as can be seen in the table, caffeine is contained in beverages and foods that children delight in consuming. Even very young infants may ingest considerable amounts of caffeine because of the practice of giving cola drinks for colic.

In considering the amount of caffeine that a young child consumes, one must take weight into account. For example, a 45-pound youngster who drinks two colas and has a chocolate bar in one day has taken in an amount of caffeine that is roughly equivalent to what a 135-pound adult would ingest from six cups of coffee.

CAFFEINE AND THE HUMAN BODY

The reason for the enormous popularity of coffee remains largely the same as it was five centuries ago—its stimulatory effects. But caffeine has additional effects on a considerable number of people, especially if they take larger-than-usual amounts. The caffeine in one or two cups of coffee may increase body temperature and elevate blood pressure, especially during stress, and because of its action on the kidneys, may result in frequent urination. Caffeine's tendency to increase metabolism in general and muscle metabolism in particular can cause mild hand tremors and impairments in the fine coordination of movement. Jitteriness and irregular heartbeat and breathing are also sometimes associated with caffeine.

Ingested caffeine, particularly when taken in the form of beverages, is absorbed rapidly. It begins to reach all organs and tissues within five minutes, and its peak effects are seen approximately half an hour after consumption. Some 12 hours later, the body has metabolized and excreted about 90 percent of the caffeine. This clearance time may explain the tremendous satisfaction many people receive from that first cup of coffee in the morning. Intriguingly, smokers tend to eliminate caffeine twice as fast as non-smokers because an enzyme that forms in the liver to cope with certain constituents of tobacco smoke also speeds up coffee metabolism. Could this be one of the reasons cigarette smokers tend to drink more coffee than nonsmokers?

The body does a very complete job of eliminating caffeine, so even if it is drunk regularly, it does not tend to accumulate in tissues and organs. This essentially total cleansing of the system leads to problems for some people. If they stop their regular caffeine intake, they start to experience withdrawal symptoms, for the body has built up a need for the drug and its absence results in discomfort. The most common symptoms are headaches that occur about 18 to 24 hours after the last dose of caffeine. Scientists have suggested that some tension headaches are in reality caffeine-withdrawal symptoms. Relief is achieved by a cup of coffee, and some researchers have noted that the headaches often occur on weekends. Individuals who have frequent cups of coffee at work may not do so on Saturday and Sunday and experience unpleasant consequences. Evidence suggests that the regular consumption of five or more cups of coffee per day may lead to some withdrawal symptoms when the caffeine intake is stopped.

Caffeine resembles other drugs in more ways than its mildly addictive properties. Regular users may develop a tolerance so that it has less effect than it used to. Thus, someone who was once stimulated by a single cup of coffee may have to increase the amount drunk to feel caffeine's stimulant effect.

Caffeine Elimination during Pregnancy

Although most people metabolize and excrete caffeine quite quickly, some groups do not. One such category is women in the later stages of pregnancy. During the first trimester, the rate of elimination does not appear to differ from the prepregnancy rate. In the second trimester, however, things start to change. By midpregnancy, caffeine clearance takes twice as long as it did before pregnancy, and a few weeks before term, the elimination rate is three times slower. Within days after giving birth, the mother clears caffeine from her system as rapidly as she did before conception.

This fluctuation in caffeine elimination during pregnancy has several implications. Most obviously, it means that the exposure of the fetus to caffeine depends not only on the amount the mother-to-be drinks but also on when she consumes it. Caffeine crosses the placenta readily; since the contents of a cup of coffee stay in the mother's and, therefore, the unborn baby's system three times longer in late than in early pregnancy, the caffeine has potentially triple the impact at the later time. Fortunately, the decrease in the elimination rate does not occur until after the first trimester, which is the time of greatest risk of gross structural abnormalities. Thus, the slowdown does not accentuate vulnerability for such aberrations. Other aspects of fetal development may, however, be subject to the consequences of the prolonged exposure.

Possibly, nature counteracts this altered biochemical response to caffeine as pregnancy proceeds. It is well known that many women lose their taste for coffee during pregnancy. In one formal study examining this question, more than a third of the subjects reduced their coffee intake during pregnancy. About half did so because of nausea associated with the beverge, and about another quarter reported that they had just lost the urge to drink coffee. Interestingly, fewer than 10 percent of the regular tea drinkers in the study reduced their intake.

THE DIFFICULTIES OF RESEARCH

To be of potential harm to a fetus, a drug must enter its circulatory system. Caffeine's physical and chemical characteristics, such as its molecular weight and solubility, allows this to occur quite easily. However, our knowledge of caffeine's influence on the course of pregnancy is very limited. One of the principal reasons is the high correlation between coffee consumption and smoking and alcohol use. It is very difficult for researchers to separate the effects of caffeine from those of these other drugs, which we know can have marked effects on the outcome of pregnancy and the development of the fetus and the newborn.

Researchers have used rats, mice, and hamsters, as well as cellular preparations, in attempts to unravel some of the questions surrounding caffeine and pregnancy. The use of animals certainly avoids any effects of alcohol and nicotine, but it presents the problem of extrapolating from the laboratory to the world of humans. The picture gleaned from about 35 studies carried out on animals and cell preparations is that caffeine can produce changes in genetic material, structural abnormalities in the fetus, and even fetal loss at dosages that seem much larger than those normally ingested by humans. However, when one takes into account the much faster rate at which small animals metabolize and eliminate caffeine, the levels of caffeine intake at which the researchers started to see fetal loss and physical abnormalities begin to fall into the range of very heavy coffee drinking (eight cups per day) among humans.

STUDIES OF PREGNANCY OUTCOMES

The West German Study

Some, although not all, of the few studies on humans support this suggestion of problems at high doses of caffeine. One of the earliest reports, from West Germany in the mid-1970s, linked high coffee consumption during pregnancy with both low birth weight and an increased risk of premature delivery. The researchers claimed that this association was independent of the cigarette and alcohol habits of mothers-to-be. Unfortunately, the reliability of these findings is questionable because of the loose way in which the researchers specified the amount of coffee drunk. Women were simply asked to categorize their consumption as "none," "seldom," or "frequent."

The Utah Study

In 1977, a United States study published some rather startling statistics on women chosen randomly from the obstetrical records of seven Utah hospitals. The fact that the subjects were obtained from a predominantly Mormon area was an important aspect of this study because the religious convictions of the Mormons make their consumption of alcohol and tobacco (and, in fact, even caffeine) relatively low compared to that of the general population of the United States. (The Utah sales of cigarettes, liquor, beer, and wine are about half the per-capita national average.) The investigators hoped that the Mormon lifestyle would make it less likely that alcohol or tobacco would confound any effects seen following caffeine use during pregnancy.

Questionnaires mailed to women who had recently given birth sought information about the caffeine-containing beverages drunk by both parents during the pregnancy. No details were gathered about the method of preparation or brand of beverage, so the researchers arrived at only a general estimate of caffeine intake. They assumed each coffee serving (no size specified) contained 75 milligrams of caffeine, tea 30, and cola 45. The investigators assessed alcohol intake simply by asking how much beer had been drunk and asked no questions about cigarette habits.

Of the almost 500 women who returned their questionnaires, 16 reported daily drinking of at least eight cups of coffee or the equivalent—600 milligrams of caffeine by the standards used in this study—while their husbands' intake averaged slightly less. Remarkably, only one of these 16 pregnancies was normal! Of the others, eight ended in spontaneous abortions in the first trimester, five in stillbirths, and two in premature births.

In these 16 families, both the mother and the father had a very high level of caffeine consumption. The researchers did not present any data from households in which the mother but not the father consumed large amounts of caffeine. However, they did describe 13 families in which the father was reported to have had an average caffeine intake equivalent to at least eight cups of coffee a day while the mother consumed less than five cups or the equivalent. The incidence of uncomplicated pregnancies in this group was much higher than in cases where both the mother and father averaged close to eight cups of coffee, but it was still half the proportion seen in families that reported no caffeine use.

Putting all these figures together led the researchers to conclude that a daily intake of caffeine equivalent to eight or more cups of coffee is associated with a substantial increase in the risk to fetal well-being and that a significant contribution to the risk factor may come from the male who consumes that much caffeine.

A number of aspects of this study can be questioned. The researchers gathered no data on cigarette habits and assessed alcohol use only in terms of beer intake. They based their findings on a small number of women. The assumption of little or no use of tobacco, alcohol, and other drugs may not be warranted. Seventy-five percent of the participants in this study were members of the Church of Jesus Christ of Latter-Day Saints, which forbids the use of not only illegal drugs, alcohol, and tobacco but also caffeine. As the risk to pregnancy was found in households in which the mother and/or father used caffeine heavily, it is quite possible that the individuals did not follow some of the other Mormon regulations on drugs.

Despite these shortcomings, this study raises a specter that must be examined. We have urgent need of careful, large-scale studies examining the possibility of fetal loss resulting from heavy caffeine use by one or both parents.

The Harvard Study

In contrast to the Utah study, a more recent project analyzed only pregnancies in which the women delivered their babies, and it found no association between coffee consumption and adverse outcomes. In 1982, a group of researchers at Harvard University interviewed 12,000 women a few days after they gave birth. The subjects were asked about their use of coffee and tea during first trimester and about their alcohol and cigarette habits throughout the pregnancy. The researchers phrased the coffee and tea questions in terms of cups per day and did not attempt accurate caffeine estimates (neither the brand nor method of preparation were determined nor were questions asked about other caffeine-containing substances).

The 5 percent of the women who reported drinking four or more cups of coffee daily were designated heavy coffee drinkers. Thus this study differed from the Utah study not only by excluding women who miscarried but also by setting the lower level of heavy use at about half the figure used in Utah. Futhermore, the Harvard work made no mention of the coffee habits of the fathers.

Like other studies of the characteristics of coffee drinkers, the Harvard research found that the frequency of smoking is greater among heavy coffee drinkers than among women who drink little or no coffee or tea—in this particular study, it was three times greater. Another characteristic of heavy coffee drinkers in this study indirectly supports the Utah findings. In previous pregnancies, these four-cups-a-day women were more likely than the others to have had serious complications, including stillbirths and spontaneous abortions. Whether this poor obstetrical history was caused by caffeine or by other factors was not investigated.

For the pregnancy just completed, however, the researchers did separate smoking and caffeine effects, a division that proved to be of critical importance. Initially, the workers compared the pregnancy outcomes of the heavy coffee drinkers with those of the remainder of the women. They found no differences in the number of stillbirths, but the heavy drinkers had a larger proportion of infants who were delivered prematurely and/or had low birth weights.

Because the Harvard researchers used a very large sample, they could separate their heavy coffee drinkers into those who had smoked during pregnancy and those who had not. Subsequent re-analysis of the data showed that the infants born to nonsmokers who were heavy coffee drinkers were indistinguishable in terms of birth weight and length of gestation from the babies born to women who had not drunk coffee. It was the smoking, either alone or in combination with the coffee, that was associated with the undesirable outcomes of pregnancy. The researchers concluded, therefore, that if the mother is a nonsmoker, four cups of coffee per day does not increase the risk for stillbirths, prematurity, or small-for-dates babies.

STUDIES OF MALFORMATIONS

A baby born with physical malformations is another adverse outcome of pregnancy. Concern that caffeine may cause such birth defects has arisen primarily from animal studies in which high doses appear to have caused malformations in offspring. About half-a-dozen studies have looked at the relationship between caffeine intake and human birth defects. Only one found any association.

The Utah study reported no abnormalities among the relatively few surviving offspring if one or both parents were heavy consumers of caffeine. Similarly, the Harvard researchers saw no increase in major or minor malformations in the offspring of heavy users.

A recent Boston study looked at the question of malformations and caffeine in a somewhat different manner. Rather than taking a large number of pregnancies and exploring the caffeine habits of the mothers who did and did not have babies with malformations, the researchers selected six of the most common birth defects and located babies born with them between 1976 and 1980 in the Boston, Philadelphia, and Toronto areas. More than 2,000 such infants were identified. Subsequently the investigators interviewed the mothers and determined their tea, coffee, and cola intake during pregnancy. As in the earlier studies, details about brands and preparation were not obtained. Coffee was assumed to contain 100 milligrams of caffeine per cup, tea 35, and cola 45. About 11 percent of the sample had ingested four cups of coffee or the equivalent daily during pregnancy, and the researchers, like those at Harvard, classified this group as the heaviest-use category. Within the levels studied, they found no evidence that the likelihood of birth defects increased with the amount of caffeine ingested.

The only study that has found an association between physical abnormalities and caffeine was a 1978 report from Belgium. In that work, researchers contrasted the caffeine use of 202 women who had malformed newborns with a control group who bore physically normal babies. A higher proportion of mothers of the infants with birth defects reported that they had drunk eight or more cups of coffee daily during pregnancy. Coffee drinking at less than this level was not found to be associated with an increased likelihood of a physical abnormality. The researchers also examined tobacco use, the age of the mother, and the number of medications taken during pregnancy—all variables that, if increased, might add to the risk for birth defects—and determined that none of them underlay the association between very heavy coffee drinking and the physical abnormalities seen in the newborn. However, the study did not consider many other potential contributing factors, including such important ones as other drug use by the mother, genetic background, and the father's drug use. These omissions plus the small number of subjects suggest that the results, as the authors themselves point out, must be viewed with caution and as preliminary. Still, it is intriguing that, this study, like the Utah study, found that eight cups of coffee was the point at which an increased risk for the unborn baby manifested itself.

Older Infants

Only one report in the scientific literature has examined the question of whether caffeine exposure during embryonic or fetal development has any measurable consequences when the baby is more than a few days old. This study was the one from the Seattle project, described in Chapter 3, that involved the examination of both mental and motor development in the eight-month-old babies of social drinkers. The information collected from the mothers about their habits during pregnancy included details of their caffeine intake. When the researchers examined the results of the tests in terms of the possible effects of prenatal caffeine exposure, in contrast to the consequences of social drinking, they noted no effects. As this study focused on alcohol consumption, it is, perhaps, not surprising that it gives very little detail about how many women, if any, had ingested really large amounts of caffeine. So whether caffeine does not have long-term effects or whether the Seattle project was not designed to assess such effects has to await further investigation.

BREAST MILK AND CAFFEINE

As we have seen, mothers-to-be, especially late in pregnancy, take a relatively long time to eliminate caffeine from their systems. Newborn babies, whether premature or full term, also have a slow rate of caffeine clearance— about 17 times slower than a normal nonpregnant adult. This fact has led some researchers to suggest that the young baby who is being breast-fed may be at risk from a possible accumulation of large amounts of caffeine. Nursing mothers may be getting caffeine not only from the usual sources of coffee, tea, and cola but also from a kind of pain reliever combined with caffeine that is sometimes specifically recommended for postpartum discomfort.

Does the caffeine from these substances get into the breast milk? The evidence is that it does, but only to a limited degree. Caffeine enters the breast milk quite quickly—within half an hour of the mother's ingesting the substance that contains it—reaches its peak concentration in about an hour, and is still present to a lesser degree two hours later. However, even at peak concentration, the quantity found in the milk is only a small percentage of the amount the nursing mother consumed. After women consumed a beverage with 150 milligrams of caffeine in it, researchers collected one litre (33 ounces) of breast milk, which is about the amount a three-week-old baby would drink in a 48-hour period; the milk contained 1.5 milligrams of caffeine. Thus, a breast-fed baby may accumulate caffeine, but the amount would be significant only if the mother regularly consumed very large amounts of caffeine-containing substances. The hitch here is that we really do not know what levels of caffeine may be potentially harmful to the young infant.

Caffeine and Apnea

A clue to this dilemma may be obtained from a surprising source—the treatment of premature babies who stop breathing. This cessation of breathing, which may last as long as 30 seconds, is termed apnea and occurs in about 25 percent of babies who weigh less than 2,500 grams. Frequent episodes of apnea can cause permanent brain damage by depriving the developing nervous system of oxygen. Caffeine has been shown, in animals and human adults, to stimulate the part of the brain that controls breathing. It also works on the human fetus; injections of it into a pregnant woman stimulate within seconds those rhythmic movements of the fetus's chest wall and diaphragm that begin in the second trimester and seem to foreshadow breathing.

Armed with this knowledge, pediatricians have used intravenous injections of caffeine to treat recurrent apnea in premature infants. The recommended dose is about 10 milligrams of caffeine for every kilogram (2.2 pounds) of the baby's weight. At that dose, no adverse effects appear to be associated with the caffeine, and higher doses do not seem to improve the likelihood of stopping the apnea. Larger doses have, however, been given on occasion; a published report listed four cases in which the caffeine injections were 3.5 to 13.0 times larger than the recommended dose. In all these cases, the infants displayed signs of caffeine overdose. They were very irritable and showed such symptoms as marked tremors, unusual uncontrolled eye movements, muscle rigidity, and very rapid respiration. The apnea and the resulting shortage of oxygen to the nervous system may have caused these symptoms, but it is interesting that they diminished over the same time required for elimination of the caffeine from the infant's body.

Caffeine administered directly into the veins of a premature baby may have quite different consequences from caffeine obtained via mother's milk, so one must be very cautious in extrapolating from the medical application to the dietary receipt. Still, the former is at least a starting point for looking at possible untoward effects of caffeine concentrations in the young infant.

As a sidelight to the topic of apnea and caffeine, it is worth noting some researchers' theorizing that the culprit and the cure may be, in part, one and the same. The speculation is that the nonbreathing episodes in the premature infants may be an expression of caffeine withdrawal. If the systems of the fetus become used to a fairly high level of caffeine during gestation, then when birth withdraws the baby from the source of the drug, the part of the nervous system controlling respiration may respond by slowing or, in an extreme case, stopping respiratory activity.

Two lines of evidence fuel this thinking. First, many newborns have caffeine present in their blood streams—not a surprising finding given the slow rate at which the mother excretes caffeine late in pregnancy and the even slower clearance rate of the baby. Second, a number of researchers have noted that apnea rarely starts immediately after birth but usually three or four days later. That three- or four-day period coincides with the time it would take the infant to excrete accumulated caffeine and begin to show signs of withdrawal, if they were to occur.

Crib death, or as doctors call it, sudden infant death syndrome (SIDS), is the tragic death of an apparently healthy infant several weeks after leaving the hospital. Whether crib death has any relationship with apnea is not known, but studies are presently underway to examine the effects of caffeine on babies who have had a near escape from SIDS. Some infants have been found in time—when they have stopped breathing but are still alive. Such infants have been identified as at risk for SIDS; whether caffeine can serve as a preventative respiratory stimulant for them is what is being explored.

CONCLUSION

In summary, the evidence from the relatively scant scientific data available on caffeine leads to the following conclusions. Daily consumption by the mother (and perhaps by the father) of eight or more cups of average-strength coffee or the equivalent (600 milligrams of caffeine) is associated with an increased risk to the unborn baby. If the caffeine intake is coupled with cigarette smoking, the level at which risk occurs is substantially lower—possibly at about four cups of coffee or the equivalent per day. Thus, excessive and what some people might term moderate use of caffeine-containing substances ought to be curtailed during pregnancy. Recalling the altered rates of excretion of caffeine as pregnancy progresses adds additional weight to that caution.

What about the other side of the coin? Is there a safe level of caffeine intake? This sort of question is one that needs many more studies before it can be answered with any degree of confidence from a scientific point of view. However, no evidence exists to date that the caffeine equivalent of one or two average cups of coffee per day increases the risk of complications for the fetus or newborn baby among women who are nonsmokers and who do not use other drugs, such as stimulants, with which caffeine may interact. It must be borne in mind that objective information is just beginning to come in, and the pregnant woman has to decide, on an individual basis, what her intake ought to be. If she decides to limit her caffeine intake, she should remember the multiple dietary and pharmaceutical sources of the drug.

If a woman was a heavy coffee, tea, or cola drinker before conceiving, she should alter her habits once she becomes pregnant. If she finds it difficult to reduce her intake of beverages, she should try drinking decaffeinated coffee or soft drinks other than cola. This caution is particularly true for the mother-to-be who finds her prepregnancy smoking habits impossible to curtail.

5   Cigarettes

Tobacco was first brought to Europe in the 16th century by explorers returning from the Americas. They had found that tobacco was widely used in North, Central, and South American cultures, playing a major role in magic and religious ceremonies. Ironically, considering today's knowledge, it was also an integral part of folk medicine with its purported curative powers used in preparations ranging from a cholera remedy to an ointment for boils.

Sailors under the command of such men as Christopher Columbus and Jacques Cartier brought tobacco seeds back to Europe, where prominent persons, such as Sir Walter Raleigh with his use of the Virginia clay pipe, rapidly made it highly popular. Almost immediately, some people realized the potential ill effects of tobacco and began campaigns against its use. Kings and even popes tried to stop its spread. However, neither moral nor health considerations seemed to discourage its use.

Back in the New World, many settlers smoked, sniffed, or chewed tobacco. Some brought the habit across with them from Europe, and others adopted it from the North American Indians. Colonial women often smoked pipes, as did the wives of both Presidents Andrew Jackson and Zachary Taylor.

The Introduction of Cigarettes

With the movement of the population from the countryside to the city around the time of the American Civil War, the role of women shifted, and tobacco use declined among females. The cigarette came into being during this period, followed by the machinery for its mass production. Although cigarettes were initially thought effeminate, their use became primarily a male habit.

Between the Civil War and World War I, smoking cigarettes gradually increased in popularity but remained an almost exclusively male custom. Cigarette use was, in part, promoted by the passage of strict antispitting laws, which sharply curtailed the practice of chewing tobacco.

Then things began to change. Women gained the right to vote, the exuberance of the Roaring Twenties swept society, and cigarette manufacturers discovered aggressive advertising. Women began smoking once more. In 1930, an estimated 2 percent of adult women smoked; today it is about 35 percent.

Currently, fewer women than men smoke, and many female smokers have habits that tend to reduce their tar and nicotine consumption—not smoking far down on the cigarette, not inhaling deeply, preferring low-tar, low-nicotine, and filtered brands. One statistic, however, is startling. Generally, in North America and elsewhere, men are giving up smoking in increasing numbers, but the percentage of women who smoke is not decreasing—in fact, it is actually increasing among 20- to 24-year-olds.

What about the smoking habits of women who are pregnant? Most investigators have found that about 25 percent of mothers-to-be smoke during pregnancy. What is striking about this figure is the relatively small number of women who give up smoking once they discover that they are pregnant. The ranks of nonsmokers increase by only 10 percent during pregnancy. Contrast this figure to the 400 percent increase in abstention from alcohol among social drinkers. The figures from cigarette smokers are dramatic evidence of the addictive properties of this habit.

THE CONSTITUENTS OF TOBACCO SMOKE

Tobacco smoke is made up of a mixture of gases and tiny droplets of solid matter, mainly tar, in which more than 1,000 different compounds have been identified.

Nicotine

Nicotine, the most active and powerful agent in cigarette smoke, is the addictive factor. A woman who is a one-pack-a-day smoker inhales this substance 60,000 times a year. Imagine having to give up anything you do so frequently. Add the fact that nicotine produces effects in the nervous system that the body begins to crave, and it is not difficult to understand why regular smokers feel a compulsion to have a cigarette in order both to experience its effects and to avoid the discomforts of its absence. Here then are the two fundamental aspects of any addictive drug—dependence plus withdrawal symptoms if it is not available. The power of nicotine addiction is seen in the fact that more than two-thirds of the people who have ever smoked still do so on a regular basis. By comparison, fewer than 15 percent of people who have ever used heroin are still addicted to that drug.

Nicotine can affect the fetus in two ways. First, it is a potent constrictor of the vascular system; the narrowing of the maternal blood vessels that supply the uterus causes a decrease in the amount of blood reaching the placenta and a consequent reduction in the supply of oxygen and nourishment available to the fetus. Second, nicotine crosses the placenta, enters the fetal circulation, and may act directly on the baby's organs.

Carbon Monoxide

A second constituent of cigarette smoke is carbon monoxide. Its effect is primarily on oxygen transport in both the mother and the fetus. During respiration, oxygen in the blood is attached to hemoglobin, an iron-containing constituent of the red blood cells. When normal hemoglobin comes in contact with tissues that require oxygen, it gives it up readily. When carbon monoxide is absorbed into the lungs from cigarette smoke, it enters the bloodstream and attaches itself to the hemoglobin. Carbon monoxide has an affinity for hemoglobin that is 200 times that of oxygen, so in the competition for whether the hemoglobin transports oxygen or carbon monoxide, the latter is a clear winner. As a result, the oxygen-carrying capacity of the red blood cells is reduced whenever an increased level of carbon monoxide is present. Levels of carbon monoxide are three times higher among smokers than among nonsmokers.

Compounding oxygen depletion in smokers, carbon monoxide also has the property of impairing the movement of oxygen from hemoglobin to the tissues of the body. Thus, the tissues of the smoker are shortchanged both because the bloodstream carries a decreased amount of oxygen and because the oxygen that is there has difficulty transferring from the red blood cells to the tissues.

Like nicotine, carbon monoxide crosses the placenta. In fact, the level of carbon monoxide in the baby's blood at delivery is nearly twice the level found in the mother's. This accumulation occurs because the baby's hemoglobin has a stronger tendency to capture carbon monoxide than does the mother's and because carbon monoxide remains in the fetal circulatory system considerably longer than in the mother's. These factors contribute to the estimate that for every cigarette the mother smokes, the fetus gets the equivalent effects of two.

Besides its nicotine and carbon monoxide effects, cigarette smoking is also associated with a reduction in vitamin B_{12} and vitamin C. Both are important for fetal well-being. Vitamin B_{12} plays a role in preventing anemia and may be affected by the small amounts of cyanide in cigarettes. Vitamin C is of vital importance for the growth of the fetus.

INVOLUNTARY SMOKING

Even nonsmokers frequently have to breathe air that contains a considerable amount of cigarette smoke. The source may be a family member (about half the married men who smoke have wives who don't), associates at work, or smokers in public places. This sort of exposure is called passive or involuntary smoking.

Little is known about such involuntary smoking and its effect on pregnancy. The amount of nicotine that is inhaled by the nonsmoker is about 1 percent of that absorbed by the actual smoker, and this small amount is not thought to have any detrimental effect on the well-being of either the mother-to-be or her baby. The reason the passive smoker inhales such a small amount of nicotine is that it does not remain in the air after being exhaled or drifting off in the smoke from the burning tip of the cigarette. Rather, nicotine, like so many other pollutants, settles out of the air rapidly.

This is not the case with carbon monoxide. It remains in the air until it is removed by ventilation, so if passive inhalation has any effect on pregnancy, it is probably via this product of smoking. There are reasons to speculate that regular involuntary smoking with its inhalation of carbon monoxide may affect the pregnant woman more than the nonpregnant woman. First, because the growing fetus takes up some of the space that would otherwise be occupied by the expanding lungs, the pregnant woman cannot get as much air as usual into her lungs. The compensatory result is a more rapid breathing. If carbon monoxide is present in the air, the faster respiration rate means inhalation of more of that gas, and the consequence is a reduction in the oxygen-carrying capacity of the red blood cells.

A second reason carbon monoxide in the air may particularly affect the mother-to-be is the increased demand for oxygen during pregnancy. The growing fetus with its developing tissues and organs needs oxygen, and its only source is the mother. Consider the heart of the fetus. It starts to function actively about ten weeks after conception, and as pregnancy continues, it contracts at 140 beats per minute. This muscular activity requires oxygen.

In addition, the altered physiology of pregnancy itself increases the oxygen demand. Consider the increased size of the woman's breasts and uterus and the special needs of her heart. A woman's heart rate increases from about 70 beats per minute to approximately 90 in pregnancy. Up goes the oxygen demand of that muscle.

Given these maternal and fetal needs plus the oxygen-depleting effects of exposure to carbon monoxide, regular involuntary smoking situations are a reasonable, although still speculative, source of concern for the pregnant woman.

THE RISK OF COMPLICATIONS OF PREGNANCY

Scientific evidence permits one to move from the speculative to the certain when considering whether smoking during pregnancy increases the risk of serious, possibly life-threatening complications. Whether one considers spontaneous abortions during early or midpregnancy, stillbirths late in pregnancy, or placental complications— all are more frequent among smoking women than among nonsmokers.

Spontaneous Abortion and Stillbirth

Investigations of the rate of spontaneous abortions have found that the incidence is as much as twice as great among regular smokers than among nonsmokers, with the risk going up with the number of cigarettes smoked. The findings persist even when researchers take into account other factors that may affect the rate of spontaneous abortion, including age, a history of previous abortions, and certain ethnic backgrounds.

The findings on stillbirths are slightly more complicated but just as certain. Women who, for one reason or another, are at risk for stillbirth increase this risk by smoking. Take black women, for example. In North America, black women have a higher incidence of stillbirths than do white women. (Most researchers believe that this difference reflects the fact that blacks are more likely than whites to be living in unfavorable socioeconomic conditions.) When one compares women who smoked and who did not smoke during pregnancy, the incidence of stillbirths is hardly different among the whites, but among blacks, smokers have a considerably higher rate. In other words, the smoking has an additive effect and significantly increases the risk of stillbirth.

Evidence that nicotine plays a role separate from carbon monoxide's in the risk to fetal well-being turned up in an unusual study from India. In a particular community in that country, about 16 percent of pregnant women chew, rather than smoke, tobacco. They keep wads of it—with a nicotine content estimated as equivalent to more than 4,000 cigarettes,—in their mouths for eight to ten hours a day. With this mode of tobacco use, only a small percentage of this vast amount of nicotine actually enters the women's system (the exact amount is not known) and no carbon monoxide is formed, so there is no competition for oxygen in the hemoglobin of the red blood cells. The Indian study found that the stillbirth rate among the women who chewed tobacco was an astounding 300 percent greater than the rate among those who did not. Nicotine is the suspected causative agent, but it is not known whether the result came from its constrictive properties on the blood vessels or its direct effect as a chemical poison on fetal tissues.

Impairment of the Placenta

As we saw in Chapter 1, for pregnancy to progress smoothly, the placenta, with its numerous complex jobs, must be a healthy, functioning organ. For this reason, it is of considerable importance to examine whether smoking can impair its life-sustaining role.

Nicotine is known to cause a temporary narrowing of the uterine blood bessels. It has been shown that smoking just one cigarette causes an immediate decrease in the flow of blood in the portion of the uterus that is joined to the placenta. This constriction disappears within 15 minutes after the cigarette has been butted out. However, the brief decrease may, if it occurs repeatedly, result in a reduction in the oxygen and nourishment that gets to the fetus and thus be responsible for some of the fetal losses reported among cigarette smokers.

It is also possible that these relatively moderate reductions in oxygen may start a chain reaction that results in a potentially fatal depletion for the fetus. Evidence accumulated over the years indicates that two placental problems appear more frequently among smokers than among nonsmokers. One, called placenta previa, is a complication in which the placenta lies over the cervix and in front of the fetus, blocking the passage. The second is abruptio placenta in which, as we saw in Chapter 3, the placenta prematurely separates either partially or completely from the wall of the uterus. Some researchers feel that the oxygen depletion associated with cigarette smoking may contribute to these serious placental complications. The repeated reduction of oxygen may disrupt normal placental-fetal communication, leading to the major placental difficulties.

Timing of the Risk

The association between smoking and fetal risk is not constant during all stages of pregnancy. The biggest increase in fetal deaths occurs between the fifth and the seventh month. During this stage of pregnancy, the fetus experiences the most rapid growth of its entire life, and the developing tissues, demand for oxygen is tremendous. Any shortage in supply would have its maximum effect during this period of great need, so the increased risk among smokers during midpregnancy is entirely consistant with the course of gestation.

SMOKING AND PHYSICAL ABNORMALITIES

According to most studies, smoking does not appear to be linked to an increased probability of gross malformations in the offspring. However, one large study, using data from 50,000 births, did find an association between the mother's cigarette habits and certain life-threatening physical abnormalities, including congenital heart defects and malfunctioning organs. Anomalies of this type are the fourth most common cause of mortality during the last few months of pregnancy and first four weeks after birth, accounting for about 9 percent of infant deaths during this time span. Given these statistics, it is not surprising that any link between cigarettes and anomalies receives wide attention in both the media and the scientific community. Many other research centers are currently conducting studies to verify the one report of such a link.

BIRTH WEIGHT

As we saw in Chapter 1, physicians use the mother's weight gain, whic reflects both her own bodily changes and the growth of the fetus, as a crude indicator of how the pregnancy is progressing. Many studies have attempted to determine whether smoking has an effect upon weight gain in pregnancy, but the results are inconclusive. Some of the workers who have found a reduction feel that it reflects a diminished food intake by the mother; others attribute it to a slowed fetal growth. Still other investigators have found no difference between smokers and nonsmokers. No reason for the inconsistency of the findings is readily apparent, and the issue still awaits resolution.

During the past 25 years, some 50 studies have pursued smoking during pregnancy and its effect upon the growth of the child. All together, they have measured the birth weights of more than 500,000 newborns.

The first thorough documentation of a relationship between smoking and birth weight was reported in 1957. A Californian investigator who examined almost 7,500 babies found that the number who were labeled as premature (defined in the study as weighing less than five and one-half pounds) was approximately double among those born to cigarette smokers compared with nonsmokers, and the probability of a premature birth rose with the number of cigarettes smoked daily.

That initial study has been followed by a host with findings whose consistency is unusual in scientific investigations. Virtually all investigators report a clear relationship between smoking mothers and lowered birth weights. Because these studies have assessed such a large number of infants, it has been possible to separate cigarette use from a host of other factors that may also reduce the birth weight, including low socioeconomic levels, particular geographic locations, certain ethnic backgrounds and cultures, older mothers-to-be, and number of previous pregnancies. Regardless of these other factors, the smoking of mothers-to-be appears to be associated independently with an increased risk of low birth weight.

Many researchers have also shown a dose-response relationship between smoking and low birth weights. For example, one study that examined 50,000 births in the early 1960s in Ontario found that the likelihood of a baby's weighing less than five and one-half pounds increased by 70 percent if the mother-to-be smoked less than a pack a day, compared to not smoking at all. If the mother smoked more than a pack a day, the probability of low birth weight jumped 160 percent compared to the nonsmokers' risk.

A causal relationship between smoking and low birth weight gains further credence from the finding that if a woman gives up smoking early in pregnancy, her baby will weigh virtually the same as infants born to nonsmokers. Finally, a study reported in 1978, which included more than 53,000 pregnancies, found that a mother who smoked during one pregnancy but not during another tended to have an infant of lower birth weight during the pregnancy in which she smoked.

Certainly, not all babies born to smokers are below the low-birth-weight figure of five and one-half pounds, and not all babies born to nonsmokers are above it. For example, in the Canadian study, 12 percent of the heavy smokers and 5 percent of the nonsmokers gave birth to infants in the low-birth-weight category. So although a woman who smokes during pregnancy dramatically increases the risk of having a low-birth-weight baby, the vast majority of women who smoke even a pack or more per day will not have such an infant. But the likelihood is that even if their babies weigh within the normal range, they will weigh less than the infants of nonsmokers. According to the information in more than 50 studies, the average difference in birth weight is approximately eight ounces, with a more marked reduction observed in the infants whose mothers who are the heavier smokers.

One might ask whether eight ounces matters. In fact, isn't it easier to deliver a smaller baby? It is true that half a pound is usually of little clinical significance. But one has to consider what caused this reduction in growth. Could the responsible mechanisms also affect more subtle aspects of the newborn, including physical and mental health?

A Direct or an Indirect Link?

Some authors feel that the link between smoking and small infants is only an indirect association, rather than a directly causal one. Their basic premise is that smokers as a whole are different from nonsmokers in more ways than their use of cigarettes. Few researchers would disagree with this claim. Fox example, as a group, smokers tend to drink more coffee and alcoholic beverages than nonsmokers. The two groups also differ in terms of work history, education, and number of previous pregnancies.

Even when these kinds of factors are discounted, however, smoking during pregnancy still has its own demonstrable effects. Those who do not accept these effects as directly caused by smoking argue that what are really being observed are the effects of the smoker as opposed to the effects of smoking. The investigation that served as the basis for this interpretation involved questioning more than 5,000 women about their smoking habits during and after recent and previous pregnancies. What was found was an eye-opener. Low birth weight occurred as often in babies born to the mothers who started smoking only after giving birth as in the infants of those women who had smoked during pregnancy. That is, women who were future smokers had newborns who did not differ in weight from the offspring of women who were current smokers. These results argue against the notion that cigarette smoking is a direct causal element in the higher incidence of low birth weight. Rather, they imply that the smaller baby results from some characteristics of the smoker herself. Possibly, factors that contribute to a woman's starting smoking may also affect the size of the baby, even if she does not actually start to smoke until after the pregnancy. In other words, cigarettes may be correlated with, rather than a direct causal factor in, low birth weight.

These results are highly controversial, and the study has been much criticized. The nonsmokers who took up the habit after pregnancy averaged several years younger than the women who smoked during pregnancy. Younger women are more likely to be having their first babies, and firstborns are generally lighter than babies born to older women who have had previous children. Moreover, the design of the study had many of the subjects being asked to recall their smoking habits during several previous pregnancies. Recollections after such a time span may well be inaccurate. Finally, the critics say, some elements that are known to influence birth weight, such as the sex of the baby and the number of previous pregnancies, were not taken into consideration.

More recent work has attempted to take at least some of these criticisms into account, but it has not settled the issue clearly. At present, all one can say is that the evidence that smoking has a direct effect on fetal growth is just too overwhelming to discount. This is not to deny that other factors that differ in smokers and nonsmokers may influence the newborn's weight. Rather, the existence of these factors and the extent of their influence on birth weight remain to be demonstrated clearly and quantified.

Small-for-Dates Babies

Do the low-birth-weight babies born to smokers tend to be premature or small-for-dates? Here the evidence is clear. Smoking during pregnancy causes a negligible reduction in the length of gestation. Studies put the average difference between smokers' and nonsmokers' pregnancies at about two days, which is not nearly enough to account for the differences in birth weight that are usually reported. The conclusion, therefore, is that smoking increases the probability of having a small-for-date infant at any gestational age—full term, preterm, and even several weeks overdue. No matter how much less or more than the normal 40-week gestational period the pregnancy may be, the birth weight of a baby born to a smoker is, on average, likely to be less than the weight of a baby of the same gestational age born to a nonsmoker.

Reduced food intake by the mother seems unlikely to be the causative factor here. Two lines of evidence converge to lead to this conclusion. Babies born to mothers known to have suffered from malnutrition during pregnancy look long and thin, but small-for-dates babies born to smoking mothers are symmetrically small. That is, everything about them is small—body length and head circumference, as well as weight. This fact suggests that the fetal growth retardation associated with smoking is not caused by a malnutrition brought about by a decreased food intake but rather by some other factor.

A second line of research has compared smokers and nonsmokers who gained the same amount of weight during pregnancy—as little as five pounds to more than forty. At every level of maternal weight gain, the investigators found that the more the mother-to-be smoked, the greater the likelihood of low birth weight, suggesting that smoking, rather than a reduction in maternal nutrition, directly affects the growth of the unborn baby.

Placental Ratio

Since the placenta is the communicating link between the mother and the unborn child, it is logical to see whether it can shed some light on the mechanisms that result in the increased frequency of small-for-dates babies, being born to smoking mothers. If placental weight is considered as a fraction of birth weight, the resulting placental ratio is higher among smoking than among nonsmoking mothers. (Actual placental weight is essentially the same for smokers and nonsmokers. But since smokers as a group do show a dose-related reduction in the birth weight of their offspring, the placental ratio increases with the amount of smoking of the mother-to-be).

This higher placental ratio may provide an important piece in the puzzle of the mechanisms underlying the relationships between smoking and small-for-dates infants. The literature reports increased placental ratios in two other situations—when births take place at high altitudes and when the pregnant woman is anemic. Both of these situations reduce the amount of oxygen carried by the mother, and it has been suggested that the relative enlargement of the placenta is a physiological response to increase the opportunity of transferring oxygen to fetus.

Thus, the research with placental ratios provides indirect evidence that smoking mothers make less oxygen available to the babies they are carrying. Coupled with the direct evidence of reduced oxygen in the blood of smoking mothers, this evidence has led most workers to conclude that the major factor in the birth weight differences of the babies of smokers and of nonsmokers is related to insufficient oxygen.

SMOKING'S EFFECTS ON NEWBORN BEHAVIOR

If an oxygen deficiency does, in fact, retard fetal growth, it may have other important consequences for the baby. In 1978, a group of researchers used the Brazelton Scale, described in Chapter 1, to compare the babies of a group of mothers who had smoked during pregnancy and a group who had not; the two groups of mothers were quite similar in other factors that are thought to affect newborn behavior. The infants were tested at four to six days of age, and some basic differences were noted. The babies of the smokers tended to be more irritable, had less ability to control their own behavior, and displayed a general lack of interest. In addition, many appeared to have impaired or reduced hearing when examined for their responsiveness to both the human voice and a bell.

In an investigation currently underway in my own research facilities in hospitals in Ottawa, the Brazelton test is also being administered to infants between two and five days of age born to smoking and nonsmoking mothers, and the results are proving similar to those of the previous work. Babies born to smokers show more irritability than and do not respond as much to sound as the infants of nonsmokers.

A clue to the link between smoking during pregnancy and newborn's altered response to sound may be found in the world of nonpregnant adults. Research has shown that impaired hearing can result from levels of carbon monoxide in the blood that are even slightly higher than normal. It has also been proposed that a major cause of hearing loss is the reduced blood flow that follows smoking. In other words, a fetus being carried by a mother who smokes is exposed to factors that are thought to influence adult hearing, and one can logically suppose that they may affect the development of the hearing system. If so, the consequence would likely be a deficiency in hearing, as noted in two studies. (It must be emphasized that neither study found the babies to be deaf; rather maternal smoking was associated with subtle impairments of the newborns' hearing. Further, no study has looked to see if these impairments are still apparent beyond a few weeks of age).

The increase in irritability and other behavior indicative of discomfort among many of the babies of maternal smokers may be related to the phenomenon of nicotine withdrawal. When adults who have been regular smokers give up cigarettes, their bodies protest as the level of nicotine in the blood falls. The symptoms are well known—the craving for a cigarette, irritability, restlessness, sleep disturbances, headaches, and impairment of concentration. Because some of the nicotine inhaled by the smoking mother-to-be passes through the placenta, the fetus's circulatory system carries its own nicotine. At birth, the baby is suddenly removed from the source of the drug. If, as appears reasonable to assume, the infant adjusts during gestation to nicotine levels in the blood, the sudden lack of the substance at birth would have consequences parallel to the withdrawal symptoms experienced by adults. (Maternal dependencies on narcotics are known to result in several days of much more severe withdrawal symptoms in the newborn.) Crying, tremors, and irritability are the only ways in which the infant can express discomfort. Underlying that distress may be the physical disturbances associated with the withdrawal of nicotine.

Our Ottawa study is revealing some additional effects. The infants of maternal smokers show consistently less habituation to repetitive stimuli, visual or auditory. The differences between the two groups of babies are marked. While the infants born to nonsmoking mothers usually stop pronounced response after four or five presentations of either light or sound, the babies born to the smokers often do not significantly reduce their startles even after nine or ten presentations. They also display many more tremors in their arms and legs, whether they are crying or not.

As we have already seen, the newborn's ability to tune out repeated, unimportant stimuli is considered an indication of a healthy, well-functioning nervous system. The finding that maternal smoking appears to be associated with an infant's inability to habituate suggests that smoking may have some subtle effect upon the fetal nervous system. The presence of more tremors than the usual may indicate the same thing.

STUDIES OF OLDER BABIES AND CHILDREN

Do the differences seen in some of the infants born to smokers persist beyond the first few days of life? As the baby gets older and older, it becomes progressively more difficult to determine the role of fetal exposure in any subsequent anomalies. Keeping in touch with children for several years and taking repeated measurements present practical problems. Investigators also face the dilemma of sorting out the effects of events during the postnatal growth of the child, many of which may influence the very things the researchers are examining, making the interpretation of results a complex matter. For these reasons, the long-term effects of smoking during pregnancy are less well documented than some of the findings described earlier.

Growth

One of the earliest studies of long-term effects tested the hypothesis that if cigarette smoke acts as a low-grade poison retarding fetal growth, the smaller babies born to smokers could be expected to grow more quickly once they were away from the influence of the smoke. Weight gain and increases in head circumference in the babies of smokers and nonsmokers were compared at six weeks, six months, and one year after birth. The growth rate in both measurements was indeed larger among the smokers' babies up to the sixth month; however, the spurt had stopped by age one, when they tended to be lighter than the children born to nonsmokers.

Other studies have followed children for several years. Their findings suggest that fetal exposure to tobacco smoke has long-lasting effects on growth, but that the effects are relatively small and become apparent only when large numbers of youngsters are examined. For example, two scientists examined data from 17,000 children—almost all the babies born in England, Scotland, and Wales in a one-week period during 1958. On average, the children of mothers who had smoked ten or more cigarettes per day during pregnancy were approximately half an inch shorter than their counterparts born to nonsmokers.

A Canadian study compared six-year-olds for weight and height, dividing the children of both smokers and nonsmokers into those who had been born prematurely, small-for-dates, and with "normal" birth weights. In all three categories, the children of nonsmoking mothers averaged approximately one-half to three-quarters of an inch taller and one to three pounds heavier than children of smoking mothers. These long-term effects were not restricted to children who had been small at birth. In fact, the most consistent differences were noted among the children who were classified as having had "normal" birth weights.

Development

Some studies have also considered the possible consequences of maternal smoking for the cognitive and motor development of the child. The researchers in my own facilities have observed that one-year-olds born to smokers consistently perform less well than age-matched infants born to nonsmokers on tests of muscular control and verbal understanding. The findings hold even when the investigators take into account the social milieus in which the babies are being raised and noncigarette drug habits during pregnancy.

Other workers have looked at the intellectual development of somewhat older children. In the previously mentioned studies of physical growth, investigators also tested cognitive traits. The British study examined reading, mathematics, and general ability when the children were 11. The scores for tests such as these are expressed in terms of the age level at which the child is performing. The children of the smokers averaged three to five months behind the other children.

In parallel fashion, the Canadian study of six-year-olds found that children born to smokers averaged scores that were consistently lower than those of their counterparts born to nonsmokers.

In all cases, the long-term effects of maternal smoking are small compared to those of other influences, such as social class and the number of other children in the family. Nevertheless, the findings do suggest a continuing effect from smoking that occurred during pregnancy.

Hyperactivity

Some researchers have also looked to see whether any behavioral abnormalities can be linked to maternal smoking habits. Although tenuous, one study suggested an association between smoking during pregnancy and a pattern of hyperactivity, which, as we have seen, is characterized by persistent restlessness and inattentiveness—a pattern of excessive activity in situations that call for the suppression of certain movements. Typically, this disorder shows itself between the ages of two and six years and begins to fade during adolescence, and because hyperactive behavior is most clearly evident in situations in which the youngster is required to be attentive and relatively still, the disorder is often first recognized in a school setting.

In testing for a relationship between hyperactivity and the effects of smoking on the fetus, the researchers compared the smoking habits during pregnancy of mothers of hyperactive children, mothers of children who were not hyperactive but were being treated at a clinic for reading difficulties, and mothers of children with no apparent disorders. Twenty hyperactive children were compared with equal numbers of children, matched for age, sex, and social class, in the other two groups. The differences in the smoking habits of the mothers of these three groups were striking and suggestive. The mothers of the hyperactive children had consumed more than twice as many cigarettes during pregnancy than the women in the other two groups. In fact, 16 out of the 20 women who had hyperactive children had smoked during pregnancy. Although the study did not report the prenatal smoking habits of the other women, one can presume, using national averages, that six to eight of each control group were smokers.

What could be the link between behavioral disorder and smoking during pregnancy? The reasoning is that slight damage to the functioning of certain parts of the brain seems to underlie hyperactivity. (In fact, some workers use the term "minimal brain dysfunction" to describe the disorder.) The researchers who conducted this smoking-hyperactivity study suggest that such damage could result from the reduced availability of oxygen that is a consequence of smoking during pregnancy.

These data must be viewed as preliminary and are, at

best, only suggestive, but the possibility that they raise certainly merits consideration and further investigation.

BREAST-FEEDING AND SMOKING

Some intriguing studies of maternal smoking concern nursing. During a woman's monthly cycles, the breasts, under the influence of hormones produced in the ovaries, develop in preparation for pregnancy. If conception does not take place, the levels of these hormones drop, menstruation follows, and the breasts return to the pre-hormonal state. When conception does occur, the production of hormones increases and the development of the breasts proceeds in preparation for lactation.

The birth of a baby sets off a series of complicated hormonal interactions in the mother that lead to the breast glands, actually producing milk. Soon after delivery—occasionally on the second day and nearly always by the third or fourth day—the breasts become larger, firmer, and sometimes somewhat painful. This is a sign that secretion of milk has begun. Sucking stimulation is a key initiator of both the production and the release of milk.

Scientists have identified more than a hundred constituents in breast milk, but its essential nutritional components are protein, sugar, salts, vitamins, minerals, and a variety of fatty compounds. The percentages of these compounds differ from individual to individual; even for a particular woman, the composition of the milk changes not only from day to day but also at various times of day. In terms of its nutritional content, breast milk is surprisingly unaffected by the mother's state of nutrition. Under-nourished women often managed to feed their babies relatively well, even during times of famine.

The quantity, as opposed to the quality, of milk depends to a large degree on the amount of fluid ingested by the mother. In addition, an estimated 1,000 calories per day are required to produce the energy used in the secretion of the milk, so a mother's intake of food ought to reflect this new demand.

Many, if not all, products ingested by the mother are excreted in breast milk in some form. Fortunately, the vast majority have clinically insignificant effects on the infant because the amounts are small. For over 50 years, scientists have known that nicotine is secreted into the milk and remains there for as much as eight hours after smoking. As one might expect, the more the mother smokes, the higher the quantity of nicotine in the milk. It is not known whether the nicotine content of the milk is essentially the same throughout a nursing session.

It is also not established whether the amount of nicotine transmitted in breast milk has any effect on the nursing baby. There have been some reports of nursing babies displaying clinical signs of mild nicotine "poisoning." These symptoms, which include restlessness, vomiting, loose stools, and an increased heart rate, were reported to lessen and then disappear as the breast-feeding mothers stopped smoking. On the other hand, many reports have found no ill-effects of nicotine in the suckling babies of smoking mothers.

Another aspect of smoking and nursing that has received some attention is whether the mother's cigarette habits affect the probability of successful breast-feeding. One study of women questioned a few days after giving birth reported that the percentage of smokers among nursing mothers was approximately a third less than among the women who were bottle feeding. Such a finding has several possible interpretations. One is that the women who are breast-feeding may be somewhat more health-conscious than those who are not, and thus less likely to smoke. Another comes from evidence that women who smoke tend to be more anxious than nonsmokers; anxiety could be the causal factor in the differences in lactation. Alternatively, smoking may interfere with lactation itself, reducing the milk supply so that not enough is available for the baby.

Several physicians have made the general observation that the incidence of an inadequate quantity of breast milk appears to be higher among smokers than among non-smokers. Unfortunately, no surveys of large numbers of carefully matched smokers and nonsmokers have specifically examined nursing habits and difficulties. One interesting report did produce data consistent with the idea of smoking's interfering with lactation. It looked at more than 500 women and the feeding patterns for their first babies. Among those mothers who breast-fed, the average number of months the women nursed was considerably smaller for smokers than for nonsmokers. But women who had given up smoking during pregnancy continued to nurse for a time similar to that of the women who had never smoked. Unfortunately, the researchers did not ask the mothers why they stopped breast-feeding, so although the study is suggestive, we cannot assume that lack of an adequate milk supply was the reason the smoking women stopped sooner.

WHEN TO STOP SMOKING?

Another issue is the timing of giving up or reducing cigarette smoking. A number of large studies have found that giving up smoking as late as the beginning of the second trimester reduces the likelihood of many adverse effects for the developing baby. A recent American study, however, disputes this finding with data suggesting that smoking even in the year before pregnancy increases the risk to the fetus. Although this issue remains to be resolved, researchers working in the area of pregnancy and smoking do agree that the best way to reduce the risk of cigarettes, affecting the unborn baby is for the mother to give up smoking as long before the birth as possible.

CONCLUSION

This chapter has summarized our present knowledge about smoking and pregnancy. There is no doubt that the components of tobacco smoke cross the placenta and enter the circulatory system of the fetus. Smoking cigarettes in pregnancy has been shown to affect adversely the fetus, the newborn, the infant, and the older child. Its potential effects range from an increased risk of life-threatening complications to a slowing of fetal growth that is later seen in reduced weight, length, and head circumference. The evidence found at birth and during the first few days of life suggests that smoking during pregnancy increases the likelihood of mild disorders of the nervous system as reflected in tremulousness, irritability, and a decreased tendency to ignore repetitive stimuli. Other consequences that appear during infancy are subtle hearing impairments and interference with nursing. Finally, some evidence suggests long-term effects—reduced physical growth, slightly poorer performance on intelligence tests, and some behavioral disorders in school-age children have all been linked to cigarette use during pregnancy.

The relationship between maternal smoking and some of these complications and adverse outcomes is not definitely established, but there is enough convincing evidence to state most emphatically that cigarette use during pregnancy cannot be regarded as medically inconsequential. The possibility of smoking's affecting the unborn child is great enough to make a very strong case for stopping the habit during pregnancy. If the health of the baby is already at risk from some other known or unknown factors, the added effect of smoking may be the straw that breaks the camel's back.

Although it is best for a woman never to have smoked or to have given up cigarettes for a considerable length of time prior to her pregnancy, it must be emphasized that almost every risk factor associated with maternal smoking appears to have a dose-response relationship. That is, the more cigarettes a woman smokes, the greater the probability that the baby will be affected. Thus, if a pregnant woman finds she cannot give up smoking entirely, a reduction in the number of cigarettes she smokes will reduce the likelihood of her habit's affecting the unborn child.

Few plants can claim as interesting and varied a history as marijuana. One of the oldest domesticated plants known to man, it has been grown for both utilitarian and intoxicating purposes.

USES OF MARIJUANA

The weedlike marijuana plant requires little more than a climate with hot summers to thrive. Like most weeds, it absorbs large amounts of nutrients from the soil and grows rapidly—up to heights of 20 feet. Depending upon the intended use of the plant, marijuana farmers use different growing strategies. The intoxicating portion is a sticky resin secreted by small hairs located around the flowers. From nature's point of view, the purpose of the resin is to protect the plant from drying out. In general, the hotter the climate, the more resin is produced. Growing the plants relatively far apart to allow more sunlight to fall on each is a procedure used to increase the resin in relatively cool climates.

The stem of the plant is covered with strong fibers that can be spun or twisted to produce hemp, which is used for cloth and rope. The production of strong fibers is best in a mild, humid climate and can be enhanced by growing the plants close together, forcing them to grow long stems.

The influence of climate on the plant was the reason that Western Europeans viewed marijuana as a source—and an important source—of fibers until the 19th century, whereas East Indians and Arabs valued it primarily for its resin and only secondarily as a source of material for cloth and rope.

Eastern Influence Spreads

European awareness of the mind-altering properties of marijuana began slowly with anecdotes brought back by adventurers to India, Africa, and Asia. The Napoleonic wars at the turn of the 19th century were a major step in spreading the word about its power to intoxicate. The French soldiers who invaded Egypt became acquainted with many aspects of life there including the use of hashish, a potent form of marijuana, and with their return to their homeland, word of its effects spread quickly.

During that age of romanticism, the famous Hashish Club of Paris came into existence. Its members, who included some of the best-known literary and artistic personages of the time, met monthly at an elegant hotel, where they sampled hashish and then retired to drawing rooms to experience its effects. Not surprisingly, Alexander Dumas, an active club member, included a hashishlike substance in the plot in one of his most popular adventure novels, *The Count of Monte Cristo*. Other members of the Hashish Club also wrote about their meetings, frequently describing their mind-altering experiences in vivid prose. These works were widely read, and the intoxicating potential of the drug soon became well known among the people of France and other European countries.

In the mid-19th century, American authors also began writing about their experiences with hashish, and it began to emerge as an important component of many plots in adventure stories. It was through this avenue, one that emphasized uncontrollable passions and considerable violence, that most Americans learned of another use for a plant that they had been harvesting for its fibers for two centuries.

Marijuana as a Medicine

At the same time that hashish was becoming known in the West for its mind-altering properties, it was also gaining a reputation for useful medicinal properties. This certainly wasn't a new notion. As early as the second century, the Chinese had mixed marijuana resin with wine as an anesthetic for surgery. In India, *bhang*, a drink made from marijuana leaves, had been used for centuries to cure fever, treat dysentery and sunstroke, and enhance the appetite.

On the other side of the world, the medicinal use of marijuana originated in the folk medicine of the peasants of Eastern Europe. Reports from the 16th century describe heating the seeds from the hemp plants until they gave off vapors that, when inhaled, relieved pains such as those of toothache. For unknown reasons, little medical knowledge spread from the peasants to urban dwellers, and the residents of the cities learned of marijuana's possible medical uses not from experience in their own countries but from travelers to the East.

In the 1840s, a Dr. O'Shaughnessy returned to England from a nine-year stint in India, where he had served as a surgeon and professor in a medical college. He described in detail the medicinal uses to which Indians put the marijuana plant. He also brought back a supply of the drug, and a large pharmaceutical company began making it commercially available. It rapidly gained a reputation among many physicians as a cure-all for a host of problems, including loss of appetite, insomnia, pain, headaches, and the withdrawal symptoms associated with narcotic and alcohol abuse. One of the first properties European doctors claimed for marijuana was an ability to increase and hasten contractions during labor and thereby hasten the birth process, an effect that had been part of Eastern European folk medicine's lore several centuries earlier.

In the contemporary United States, the medical profession became aware of the writings of the Europeans, and some physicians began prescribing marijuana for their patients. By the 1850s, medical texts listed the drug as a recommended treatment for a wide array of disorders similar to the list proposed in Europe. However, marijuana as a remedy did not gain much popularity in the States, where practitioners identifed numerous problems in its use, including the difficulty of obtaining marijuana with a consistent amount of active ingredients, the wide range of individual reactions to the same quantity of the substance, the slow-acting nature of the drug, and, the need to administer it orally, rather than by injection, because it is insoluble in water.

An ironic incident came from the search for the medical properties of marijuana. At the turn of the century, the United States government planted marijuana in order to have a supply with which to experiment. The cultivation was stopped after only a few years because of the increasing opinion that the plant's mind-altering properties were an evil phenomenon. The fields where the marijuana was grown are today the site of the Pentagon.

REGULATION OF MARIJUANA

Throughout the centuries, most of the societies that have included marijuana in their mind-altering paraphernalia have had laws designed to curtail its use. The basis for such edicts has generally been the belief that the drug had a potential for unleashing violent and/or sexual passions among habitual users. In the United States, lawmakers acted relatively recently. Not until the 1930s did the government launch a propaganda campaign against the perceived threat to American society. The Federal Bureau of Narcotics undertook "educational campaigns" that, by current advertising standards, appear almost ludicrous in their extreme nature, and various organizations put out posters to warn the population about the drug's dangers.

Today marijuana is not usually portrayed in lurid prose, but its use still engenders considerable passion among both its opponents and proponents. This book is not the place to jump into that debate. One consequence of the heated controversy does, however, bear on the topic of this book. Unfortunately, most statements claiming that marijuana damages or is harmless to the unborn babe are more likely to reflect the author's biases, beliefs, and even passions rather than his or her knowledge of objective data on the topic. In fact, the information available is too sparse to permit definitive, dogmatic conclusions.

THE HUMAN BODY AND MARIJUANA

Having said this, let us consider our present knowledge of marijuana. Chemically, it comprises several compounds; the principle mind-altering constituent has the tongue-twisting formal name of 1-delta-9-transtetrahydrocannabinol. Mercifully, this can be abbreviated to Δ^9-THC or, for less-than-purists, just THC, and that's what I call it in the rest of the chapter.

When marijuana is smoked, the effects of THC are felt within five minutes of the first inhalation, with the peak effects reached in half an hour to an hour. In a healthy adult, the liver breaks down the THC in a series of chemical reactions, with the final products excreted in the feces and, to a lesser degree, the urine.

Compared to other "soft" drugs, marijuana is eliminated from the body relatively slowly, with traces being found as long as eight days after use. The fact that marijuana clearance takes so long has important implications for a regular user. If the liver does not have time to clear the body before the next joint is lit, the drug's constituents can accumulate in various tissues. The greater the accumulation, the longer it takes to clear the system when drug use is stopped.

Circulation and Accumulation

Where does ingested marijuana go in the body? As a general rule, the largest amounts of the drug appear in the parts of the body that have the most abundant blood supply —the liver, the lungs, the kidneys, and, in the pregnant woman, the placenta. There is one interesting exception— the brain. In adults, relatively small amounts of marijuana constituents enter this three-pound organ in spite of its receiving about 20 percent of the blood flow from the heart. We do not know why the brain receives only limited amounts of the drug. A partial answer may lie in the protective mechanism known as the blood-brain barrier, which prevents many potentially toxic substances from passing from the circulatory system into the brain tissue.

This barrier undoubtedy blocks some marijuana constituents, although its role with THC is uncertain. Before it is broken down by the liver, the THC in marijuana, unlike the drugs discussed in the previous chapters, is absorbed by and dissolved in fat cells, which are present in virtually all bodily tissue. Certainly, the fat cells in blood, which are termed lipoproteins, absorb and circulate THC, and lipoproteins and the substances they transport cross the blood-brain barrier quite readily. Thus THC ought to be able to enter the brain tissue. On the other hand, when the constituents of marijuana, including THC, are broken down by the liver, the metabolized products that circulate in the blood are no longer soluble in fat and so are not carried by the lipoproteins. This change may limit the amount of THC that crosses the barrier and enters the brain.

Scientists have not firmly established whether it is this mechanism or some other system that partially protects the brain from THC. Whatever the answer, a sufficient quantity ends up in that structure to cause the perceptual and behavioral changes associated with a marijuana high.

The fact that marijuana constituents are fat soluble has important implications for the length of time the drug remains in the body. When fat tissue absorbs a substance, the body has difficulty dislodging it. This is the main reason marijuana constituents remain in various systems and organs for such an unusual length of time.

Accumulation in Breast Milk

The attraction between marijuana and fatty tissue has an important ramification for the nursing mother. The tissues that make up the breasts are largely fat. If they contain marijuana constituents, the milk produced will also likely contain some, which will be passed on to the infant.

Researchers have studied THC in animals by assessing the milk produced by ewes and rodents. The investigators gave lactating females THC that had been "labeled" with a radioactive molecule. (This procedure does not alter the effect of THC nor, because of the very low amount of radioactivity involved, does it affect the animal. It does, however, permit the researcher to trace the THC as it moves through the organs and systems of the recipient animal.) Using this procedure, researchers have seen clearly that the drug does enters the milk and is transferred from the lactating animal to the suckling offspring. There is no reason to suppose that the process would be any different for human beings.

The exposure of the suckling human infant to marijuana constituents may be of significance. As described in Chapter 1, the human brain undergoes a period of rapid growth from about ten weeks before birth until almost two years afterward. This brain growth spurt occurs in all mammals, but the timing relative to the birth differs among species. Take, for example, two of the most widely used laboratory animals: in the guinea pig, the spurt occurs entirely before birth, while in the rat, it occurs entirely afterward. The spurt for humans is in between these two extremes. During the spurt, the developing brain is particularly vulnerable to damage, in terms of both growth and function. For the human baby, a considerable portion of the vulnerable period coincides with the nursing period, so potential harmful substances that may enter the milk pose a risk.

No data have been reported on the consequences of exposing a human infant to marijuana constituents via milk during the first months of life, so no definitive statements can be made as to whether there are any effects. But given the indisputable facts that the brain is going through formative development at this age and that constituents of marijuana can accumulate in breast milk, the marijuana-smoking mother who is nursing ought to be fully aware that she is exposing her young baby to a drug that has mind-altering effects in the much larger adult.

Accumulation in the Placenta

After radio-labeled THC is administered to pregnant animals, the largest amount of radioactivity is found in the placenta. This concentration is not particularly surprising as this structure has such a rich blood supply. What is somewhat surprising is that relatively little of the drug actually crosses the placenta to the fetus. The placenta does, in this case, act as a partial barrier. Nevertheless, some THC does cross and enters the fetus's organs and systems. For unknown reasons, the highest levels are found in the fetal nervous system.

Whether humans follow the same pattern is not known at this time, but the animal data is highly suggestive. It is also worth noting that the blood-brain barrier is essentially nonexistent until a few weeks after birth. Its absence may add to the vulnerability of the brain of the fetus and the very young infant.

STUDIES OF PREGNANCY OUTCOMES AND
PHYSICAL MALFORMATIONS

About 30 studies using a variety of animal species have been undertaken to determine whether marijuana or THC poses a risk to the fetus in terms of either survival or physical malformations. The vast majority of these studies suggest that deaths and malformations do not increase until quite a large quantity of the drug is administered. With rhesus monkeys, for example, levels estimated as roughly equivalent to 16 joints per day produced a pregnancy loss four times higher than expected. Notice that although this dose of marijuana is high, it is within the range of human use. This study did not find increased malformations. Others have observed them but at doses of marijuana that were well beyond those ingested by humans.

But these are animal studies. To generalize to pregnant women is an enormous jump, one that has to be made with extreme caution. The animal work serves as a guideline. It helps to focus on what questions and cautions ought to be applied to the human situation. At this stage all we can say is that for nonhuman mammals marijuana at high doses definitely poses a risk to the survival of the fetus. We do not know what the corresponding level is in humans, but all signs suggests that a risk factor exists at *some* level.

Moreover, the human situation is infinitely more complex than that of an animal study. Any risk that marijuana imposes may interact with the risk imposed by other life-style habits that often accompany the drug's use. What about marijuana with alcohol? Marijuana with tobacco? What about the combination of the drug and a poor diet? This last possibility has been looked at, although only in animal research. In my own laboratory we exposed pregnant rats to an amount of marijuana smoke roughly equivalent to six joints per day in human terms; no increase in fetal deaths was seen. Neither did a protein-deficient diet result in fetal loss. But when the marijuana treatment was combined with the poor diet, the number of stillbirths increased significantly. The additive effect of the drug *and* the protein deficiency was sufficient to cause the deaths. Again, applicability to the human situation remains to be determined, but it bears serious investigation because many women have a life-style that involves both marijuana usage and inadequate diet. Together the two factors may pose a greater risk than does each individually.

The Need for More Research

The absence of objective data on marijuana and pregnancy is difficult to understand when one considers the extent of the use of the drug. By the end of the 1970s, 43 million Americans had tried smoking it, and as many as 16 million were using it currently. Although the majority of users are males, the percentage of females who use it appears to be increasing steadily. And the age groups in which the increase is concentrated are late adolescence and young adulthood—those that are also the most likely for having children. According to recent U.S. government statistics, the usage rate is approximately 10 percent among women between 18 and 25 years of age.

In spite of the large number of women who may be placing their unborn children at risk if marijuana does have adverse effects in pregnancy, scientific work in this area has been almost nonexistent. In part, this lack reflects the difficulties of conducting research and gathering information on a substance that is illegal. It also reflects the lack of public pressure (and thus research funding) for answers to this issue. In contrast to the multitude of studies, involving several hundred thousand babies, that have focused on the potential deleterious consequences of alcohol and cigarettes in pregnancy, only two reports have appeared in which marijuana's effects are a key topic. Each was based on one woman. Each of the two subjects had used marijuana during pregnancy, but they had also used other drugs, including

LSD. In both cases, the babies had abnormalities in the bone structures of the hands, but the women's polydrug habits make it impossible to come to any conclusion, however tentative, about marijuana's role in producing the physical abnormality.

It seems reasonable to suppose that marijuana does not have a very marked effect on spontaneous abortion rates, stillbirths, or congenital abnormalities. If a clear cause-and-effect relationship existed, physicians would have noted and reported it. Since the thalidomide tragedy, the medical profession has become acutely sensitive to the problem of protecting the unborn child from use by the mother-to-be of any substance with potential adverse effects. If, however, marijuana use has a risk factor that is not very dramatic but still exists, it will be difficult to identify. Carefully monitered studies of many thousands of pregnancies are necessary to establish what risk, if any, exists. Large numbers are also needed to separate the potential adverse effects of marijuana from risks that may accompany personal characteristics and other life-style habits of the women who use the drug.

EFFECTS: THE OTTAWA STUDY

Of course, marijuana use during pregnancy may have effects other than the extreme consequences of producing death or gross abnormalities in the unborn baby. Does it affect the growth of the fetus, the length of gestation, or the behavior of the infant after birth? The complete lack of information pertaining to these sorts of questions prompted me, Dr. R. Knights, who is an internationally known psychologist specializing in young children's learning problems, and several obstetricians to undertake a long-term investigation of the consequences of the use of marijuana and other drugs during pregnancy. In the summer of 1978, the research team was put together with two primary objectives: to establish a picture of the percentage of women who use marijuana, alcohol, and cigarettes before or during pregnancy, and to examine the effects of these drugs on their babies at birth and as they get older.

To gather subjects for the study, women visiting their obstetricians are given a short letter that describes the purpose of the project. In the letter and following discussions, we point out that all pregnant women, whether they use any marijuana, cigarettes, or alcohol, are of equal interest to us. If we are to draw conclusions about, say, marijuana, we can do so only by comparing women who are alike in as many respects as possible except for their use of that drug. So, for example, if one 25-year-old smokes marijuana and a package of cigarettes a day and also drinks two beers a night, we would like to be able to compare her pregnancy and baby to those of another woman in her mid-20s who doesn't use marijuana but does smoke cigarettes and drink alcohol in the same amounts.

If a mother-to-be is interested in participating in the study, an interview is set up, usually at her home. Here we ask detailed questions about her health (both presently and before the pregnancy), history of previous pregnancies, nutritional intake, and past and present drug use. The women are interviewed once during each trimester.

What we have found on the basis of about 600 women and their babies has been quite revealing. About 80 percent did not use any marijuana in the year before pregnancy and about 7 percent smoked it on a regular basis during that period. After becoming pregnant, the nonusers rose to about 90 percent and regular users declined to about 4 percent. Three-quarters of the regular users smoked at least six joints per week during pregnancy. For descriptive purposes, we have called these women heavy users.

As a group, the heavy users have a number of, characteristics that differ from the nonusers, and occasional users. The heavy users tend to be in their early to middle 20s, in contrast to the late 20s of the other mothers-to-be. The heavy users are also more likely to have less formal education and tend to smoke more cigarettes and to drink more alcohol.

Findings on Pregnancy

Because of the relatively small number of babies born so far in this study, we are not able to state whether marijuana is associated with any increased risk for miscarriage, spontaneous abortion, or stillbirth. In terms of complications at birth or the type of presentation of birth, we have found no differences between the heavy marijuana users and the rest of the women.

What we have noticed, however, is that the heavy users have slightly shortened pregnancies—usually about one to two weeks less than those of women who do not use the drug. When gestational age is taken into account, the newborns marijuana users do not exhibit unusually low birth weights. This finding is the opposite of what we and others have found with cigarettes. As described in Chapter 5, cigarette smoking during pregnancy is associated with a lowered birth weight but not a shortened gestation period. Our "marijuana babies" show no evidence of fetal growth retardation, but they are born slightly sooner.

Another of our interesting findings at birth relates to labor itself. As already mentioned, marijuana has been used historically to increase and hasten labor contractions. In our study, a number of marijuana users who smoked very late in pregnancy reported that the drug appeared to have triggered labor. It began within an hour of using marijuana, and it started suddenly, vigorously, and with relatively little time between contractions. Although anecdotal reports are certainly not enough to prove the case, these observations coupled with the European folk tradition are certainly intriguing.

Findings in Newborns

The newborn babies of the heavy marijuana users in our study do not seem to differ physically from the other infants on the Apgar test given at one and five minutes after birth. At about four days of age, the babies are tested for their capacity to interact with stimuli in the environment using the Brazelton Neonatal Assessment Scale. Those born to the heavy marijuana users respond and habituate to sound in the same fashion as those born to nonusers. However, it is a different story when light is used as a stimulus. The infants of the heavy marijuana users are, in general, less responsive to a light shone in their eyes, and after they do respond, they tend to be less able to habituate to the repeated stimulus. The differences between the two groups of babies are quite marked. So far, among the infants born to the heavy marijuana users, 75 percent have either responded very weakly or failed to habituate, while 16 percent of nonusers' babies have behaved in a similar manner.

A few points have to be made about this altered visual response in many of the infants of the heavy users. First, the babies are not blind in any sense of the word. Rather, they have some altered responsiveness to light. Second, the same testing procedure has found a similar state of affairs among babies born to mothers who have used narcotics during pregnancy. In the latter case, the altered visual functioning is thought to be a symptom of narcotic withdrawal in the newborn. This hypothesis raises the possibility that the similar behavior in the infants born to heavy marijuana users may also reflect a form of withdrawal. Once born, they no longer have marijuana being pumped into their system. Most researchers have failed to find any sort of physical withdrawal symptoms associated with adults' stopping marijuana use, but, of course, the situation may be quite different for the fetus and the newborn.

Third, a study using rhesus monkeys has noted behavior consistent with our findings in human babies. In the animal study, the investigators gave monkeys THC before and during pregnancy and throughout the nursing period. The offspring were examined at one and two years of age for many kinds of behavior, including general activity, problem solving, responsiveness to environmental events, and social interaction. The principle category of behavior that distinguished the THC offspring from the others was visual attentiveness—in particular, the ability to habituate to visual stimuli. The similarity to our findings in humans is striking.

Visual behavior is not the only way in which our marijuana babies differ from the rest of the newborns. We also use the Brazelton test to rate the infants' general characteristics, including muscular strength, irritability, alertness, tremors, startles in reaction to unexpected stimuli, unelicited startles, the extent of crying, and the ease with which they can be consoled. We are finding that the marijuana babies consistently display many more tremors in their arms, legs, and lower jaw than do the infants of nonusers. These tremors, which are often pronounced, occur both when the infants are crying and when they are not. In parallel fashion, the marijuana babies also tend to display more startles in the absence of an obvious external cause, and their startles to an unexpected noise or light are much more marked and longer-lasting than those of the babies of nonusers. No differences have been seen in the other types of behavior examined.

The increase in tremors and startles can be interpreted in at least two ways. Like the altered visual responsiveness, exaggerated tremors and startles are seen in babies known to be undergoing narcotic withdrawal, so this behavior in our study may be further sign of marijuana withdrawal. Increased tremors and startles can also indicate an immature nervous system, one that has not developed to the extent expected by the time the baby is born. It is possible that fetal exposure to marijuana results in slow development of the nervous system. Further work is underway to determine whether one of these alternatives or some other factor may underlie these unusual characteristics in the very young infants of heavy marijuana users.

Tests of Older Babies

When we test the babies again at nine and thirty days of age, most still exhibit tremors and exaggerated responses to stimuli, although not as markedly as at four days of age. Similarly, the decreased visual responsiveness persists, but it is not as apparent as that observed when the babies are younger.

We have already tested a few babies at six months or more for motor and mental development and general behavior and found no striking effects associated with marijuana exposure during fetal development. But these are very preliminary results. It is too soon to say whether the abnormalities present at birth are overcome or compensated for with maturity or whether long-term effects exist but are of such a subtle nature that many more children will have to be tested before a risk factor can be identified.

CONCLUSION

Clearly, only the very first steps have been taken in determining the consquences of marijuana use during pregnancy. The nature of marijuana is such that the body cannot be rid of it easily. As the constituents of the drug travel in the mother's bloodstream, some are likely to cross the placenta and enter the circulatory and nervous systems of the fetus. We do not know what amount, if any, of marijuana can be used without risking the well-being of the baby, but clearly, regular daily use is associated with measurable alterations in the behavior of newborns. No data is yet available on the long-term ramifications nor have we gathered enough information to speculate on whether giving up marijuana some time during pregnancy decreases the effects seen in the newborn.

Faced with this paucity of information, the woman who uses marijuana and who is considering having a baby must recognize that she is gambling at high stakes. The odds of adversely affecting the baby are not known, but all lines of evidence from animal research and our limited human data suggest that some risk is present.

Finally, what about the father? If so little is known about the effect of marijuana use by the mother, it is not hard to predict a lack of information about the consequences on pregnancy of regular use by the male. Physicians have not reported any increase in fetal loss or physical anomalies that appears to be associated with male marijuana use. But this is a risky state of affairs on which to base a decision. Anecdotal reports (or a lack of them) are not the same as objective, follow-up studies of pregnancies. These still have to be done before any definitive statement can be made.

7   Nonprescription and prescription medicines

About a hundred years ago, Sir William Osler, one of the foremost physicians of the time, remarked, "The desire to take medicine is, perhaps, the greatest feature which distinguishes man from animals." His statement has become even more true in the past decade or two.

In 1970, doctors wrote a total of 1.3 billion prescriptions for drugs in the United States. Two years later this figure had doubled. The most recent estimate is more than 3 billion. The use of nonprescription (over-the-counter) drugs is also very common, although the absence of records means that its extent cannot be known as accurately. Even the number of available *types* of over-the-counter medications is staggering. The estimates range from 100,000 to 500,000, including antacids for upset stomachs, minor painkillers, vitamins, cough medicines, laxatives, and so on and so on.

To realize the pervasiveness of drugs in the modern environment, simply ask yourself how many drugs are in your medicine cabinet and elsewhere around the house. If yours is an average family, the number is approximately 30 —five prescription drugs and twenty-five over-the-counter medicines. And chances are that you can't name a large proportion of your household's medicines without looking and that one or two of them are in unlabeled bottles or containers.

Like other North Americans, pregnant women take medicine in large and increasing quantities. Several surveys conducted in the 1960s found that women took an average of five different medicines during pregnancy; by the 1970s, it had risen to approximately nine. One survey showed that 80 percent of the medicines were taken without a doctor's supervision or knowledge. More than half the pregnant women in one Houston study had ingested Aspirin and vitamin supplements, while more than 20 percent had taken sedatives.

The Lessons of the Thalidomide Tragedy

Before 1961, scientific work examining the effects of drugs on the fetus was largely devoted to determining the effects of anesthetics and medications given at the time of delivery. Then the thalidomide tragedy occurred, and concern immediately arose that other, previously unsuspected drugs might also be affecting the unborn.

The pivotal nature of thalidomide in changing our way of thinking about ingested substances makes it worthwhile to trace how this drug came to be taken by thousands of unsuspecting pregnant women in Europe, Canada, South America, and Australia.

Thalidomide, which became available in the late 1950s, was marketed as a tranquilizer for adults. It was effective and had no unpleasant aftereffects. It was also unusually safe in terms of the risk of overdose; the estimate of a fatal amount, based on reports of attempted suicides who had recovered after taking enormous quantities, was estimated to be about 140 times larger than the typical therapeutic dose.

This combination of apparent safety and medicinal value led to the drug's being recommended for use by pregnant women as a sedative for anxiety. Soon after there was an increase in the number of infants born with a shortening or complete absence of limbs.

Two facts combined to alert physicians to the fact that the malformations might have an external cause. First, this kind of physical anomaly had been extremely rare, seen in only one in half a million births. Second, the marked increases appeared simultaneously in many parts of the world. Yet the rise was not sharp in the United States, where the Food and Drug Administration was still testing the tranquilizer and had not licensed it for sale. Investigation showed that the malformations were appearing wherever thalidomide was marketed, and it was established that in virtually every case the mother had taken the drug between the third and eighth weeks of pregnancy. Although the detective work proceeded relatively quickly, as many as 10,000 infants may have been affected worldwide before the drug was removed from the market.

Besides focusing attention on the potential dangers of introducing foreign substances into the body during pregnancy, the thalidomide tragedy provided a strikingly clear example of how the timing of ingestion plays a critical role in a substance's effect on the developing child. When thalidomide was taken 35 or 36 days after the last menstrual period (at approximately 21 to 22 days' gestation), the babies were born with no ears. Women who ingested the drug three to five days later had babies with no arms or severely shortened ones. Those who took the tranquilizer a day or two later had infants with similar defects of the legs. The period of sensitivity to thalidomide ended 48 to 50 days after the last menstrual period.

One reason for the thalidomide tragedy was the failure of research on animals to predict the effect on humans. The drug had produced no abnormalities in pregnant rats. (Later studies did show that the rat is sensitive to thalidomide, but only on day 12 of gestation.) Unfortunately, thalidomide, like some other drugs, is more damaging in some species than in others. This discovery simply emphasizes the fact that although animal research is essential in drug research, only humans are reliable models for definitive assessments. The thalidomide example also highlights the fact that a drug that has no adverse effects on the mother may have very serious consequences for her unborn baby.

The identification of thalidomide as the causative factor in this particular malformation was possible because of the striking nature of the anomaly and because of the explosive increase in the frequency of occurrence. The problem of linking cause and effect is much more difficult in less dramatic situations. Take, for example, an attempt to evaluate the possible deleterious effects on the fetus of a relatively common medicine. The very fact that it is in everyday use is evidence that any adverse effect is not dramatic; if it were, it would have been detected long ago. If any effect exists, it is subtle and probably occurs in relatively few instances.

Noting subtle or infrequent effects requires careful observations of large numbers of pregnancies. Records must be kept on complications of pregnancy, spontaneous abortions, stillbirths, malformations, and unusual behavior at birth. Even if the researcher can show a relationship between the drug and some adverse outcome, causality may remain unproved. One extremely difficult problem is separating the effect of a particular medicine from that of the condition for which it was taken. For example, if a mother-to-be takes a drug to combat a high fever, the cause of a later complication in the pregnancy may be the drug, the fever, or the combination—or some totally unrelated factor.

Given the difficulties of research plus the tremendous number of medicines on the market (and new ones appear all the time), it is impossible for all to be tested adequately for potential effects on the unborn baby. Nevertheless, considerable research has been done during the past two decades.

In this chapter I summarize the conclusions of researchers concerning some of the most widely used medicines, over-the-counter and prescription.

NONPRESCRIPTION DRUGS

Antacids

Antacids are usually taken in response to a burning sensation just behind the lower part of the breastbone. Commonly called heartburn, this is not a serious condition, but it is not pleasant. Heartburn is relatively more common during pregacy than at other times because of the pressure on the stomach from the growing uterus coupled with a hormonally controlled increased relaxation of the muscle that normally stops stomach juice from flowing upward.

The principal concern about the use of antacids during pregnancy pertains to the sodium that some, but not all, brands contain (usually in the form of sodium bicarbonate). Researchers believe that prolonged use of these antacids is not advisable during pregnancy because the fetus, with its immature kidneys, has difficulty ridding itself of the sodium. As the chemical builds up, its body tries to counteract the effect by retaining fluid. If this situation is carried to excess, the consequences can be extremely dangerous.

Antacids that contain no sodium compounds do not appear to have any harmful effects on the fetus if used according to the directions on the package.

Painkillers

Pregnant women often take mild pain remedies, which doctors refer to as analgesics, to treat such symptoms as headache, backache, colds, and fevers. These painkillers usually contain one of two drugs—acetylsalicyclic acid (also known as ASA) and acetaminiphen. Nearly 50,000 over-the-counter brands contain one of these drugs as a primary ingredient, and Americans alone swallow an estimated 50 million doses of them each day. Clearly, for many, many individuals, they have become part of a life-style, something to be taken almost automatically for a wide variety of ailments, present or anticipated.

Medicines containing acetylsalicyclic acid (ASA) were developed at the end of the last century and today include such products as Aspirin, Bufferin, and Anacin. They are undoubtedly effective in relieving moderate aches and pains, reducing fever, and controlling the kind of inflammation that accompanies rheumatic diseases. They also have several undesirable side effects, including irritating portions of the digestive tract and, importantly for pregnant women, descreasing the blood's ability to clot.

The more recently developed acetaminophen-containing preparations, such as Tylenol and Atasol, are effective remedies for minor pains, but they lack the anti-inflammatory properties of ASA. Acetaminophen also does not produce the propensity for increased bleeding that is associated with ASA.

Remedies containing ASA have been the over-the-counter medications most extensively studied for pregnancy risk. In the late 1960s, three European studies involved interviewing a total of approximately a thousand mothers who had given birth to malformed babies. The mothers were asked about their use in pregnancy of medication containing ASA, and the results indicated that the use of such drugs was considerably higher among these women compared to others who had given birth to normal infants. However, although these findings are superficially very suggestive, they are, in fact, rather inconclusive because the studies did not always report a number of critical factors, including the reasons the women had taken ASA, their general health, and the incidence of anomalies in their families.

More recent work used a different approach. Australian researchers identified women who were heavy ASA users during pregnancy and followed them up after they gave birth. The findings were an incidence of malformations among the babies of these women that was slightly higher than among the infants born those who used little or no ASA, but again interpretation is difficult. First, the study included only 144 heavy users. Furthermore, these women were also heavier cigarette smokers than their counterparts. The report did not discuss the possible influence of cigarettes on its findings, although, as described in Chapter 5, smoking during pregnancy may be linked with an increased risk of anomalies.

In fact, the study that reported an association between the mother's cigarette habits and physical abnormalities also examined the use of aspirin during pregnancy and the risk of malformation. This American study considered more than 50,000 pregnancies. Almost two-thirds of the women reported using ASA at some time during pregnancy, but the researchers failed to find any association between this medication and fetal malformation.

Most researchers, currently think that if the mother is not using other drugs that contribute to the likelihood of physical anomalies, ASA in the recommended dosage does not significantly increase the risk of cogenital malformations.

ASA is not viewed quite so benignly, however, when it comes to other types of risk during pregnancy. Since 1966, scientists have known it interferes with the blood's ability to clot, so that if any bleeding occurs, it continues for a prolonged period of time. These effects are seen at standard medical doses and, somewhat surprisingly, continue for up to a week after the last dose. This phenomenon has ramifications for both the pregnant woman and the baby she is carrying. Studies have associated the use of ASA in the third trimester with a greater-than-normal loss of blood at delivery, and women who used ASA regularly during the last month or so of pregnancy have been shown to require blood transfusions during delivery much more frequently than do nonusers.

For the fetus and newborn, the maternal intake of ASA may have even more serious consequences. The drug crosses the placenta freely, and if the mother has taken it relatively soon before giving birth, it is found in the infant's bloodstream. The mechanism for the metabolism of acetylsali-cyclic acid barely functions in the fetus and newborn, and thus the drug remains longer in this blood than it does in the blood of an adult. For example, one study reported a marked deficit in the blood-clotting ability of newborns whose mothers had ingested ASA two weeks before delivery.

If the birth is a difficult one or if the baby is premature, infantile bleeding is a real possibility, particularly in the region of the brain, and the likelihood of a hemorrhage increases markedly if the baby's bloodstream contains ASA. In such a case, the hemorrhage may also be more extensive. The seriousness of this problem is underlined by studies using autopsies of babies who died within a few weeks of birth. As many as three-quarters of the deaths involved bleeding of the central nervous system.

ASA has also been found to increase the average length of gestation and to prolong labour. It is suspected of doing this by interfering with the body's production of chemicals that stimulate the contraction of the uterus.

Taken together, the side effects of ASA are sufficient to suggest strongly that women should not ingest medi-cines containing it during the last three months of preg-nancy. If medication is needed for pain relief, remedies containing acetaminophen are a safer choice. Of course, all drugs must be used with caution during pregnancy, and because of their relative newness, painkillers based on acetaminophen have not been tested as thoroughly as ASA. However, the work to date, including tests for blood-related complications, has not indicted any adverse effects for mother or child.

VITAMINS

Adequate quantities of vitamins are necessary for the normal development and health of the ftus, but this does not mean that vitamins ought to be gobbled down in preg-nancy as routinely as three meals a day. Despite nature's high demand for vitamins during pregnancy, most mothers-to-be do not require vitamins in addition to an adequate, well-balanced diet.

Vitamins can be divided into those that are soluble in fat and those that are soluble in water. The former are stored principally in the liver and are released when the body requires them. Vitamins A, D, E, and K are in this category. A deficiency in these fat-soluble vitamins is rare, but overdosage is a potential danger as relatively little of them is excreted in the urine.

The water-soluble vitamins include the B-complex vitamins, ascorbic acid, and folic acid. They are readily excreted in urine, and although the body stores them in appreciable amounts, they are not kept in reserve to the same degree as are the fat-soluble vitamins. This makes overdosage less likely.

Vitamin A

Several physiological functions are associated with vitamin A. It is needed for vision, growth, and development of tissue and bone. In the mother-to-be, the level of vitamin A decreases early in pregnancy, rises in late pregnancy, falls during labor, and increases again after the birth.

Water-soluble vitamins, of which Vitamin A is one, are measured in International Units (IU). The recommended daily amount of Vitamin A for a pregnant woman is 6,000 IU, which is 25 percent more than the amount recommended for women who are not pregnant. The additional allotment is to meet the needs of the fetus and is usually obtained from the diet. The liver of the mother stores the vitamin and releases it as demand for it increases. Rarely is there a need for a vitamin-A supplement because it is obtained from butter, cheese, egg yolks, and many vegetables.

Some food faddists recommend massive doses of vitamin A, but this should be avoided, particularly during pregnancy. Data from both animal and human studies link fetal exposure to megadoses of vitamin A with anomalies of the nervous system and kidneys.

Vitamin D

Vitamin D, which is obtained from the action of sunlight on the skin, is important in the formation of bones and in maintaining a suitable level of calcium. Too much vitamin D can upset the calcium balance; such an occurance during pregnancy can lead to the baby's developing serious skeletal problems and being mentally retarded. The recommended daily amount of this vitamin is 400 IU for both pregnant and nonpregnant women.

Vitamin E

Vitamin E, which is found in cereals, egg yolks, and beef liver, plays a role in normal muscular development and a number of biochemical processes in the body. Pregnant women who are eating normal diets need no supplement. The recommended dose is 30 IU daily for pregnant women, 20 IU for nonpregnant women.

Vitamin K

Vitamin K, found in leafy green vegetables and cereals, is important in the development of the blood-clotting mechanism. Unless prescribed by a physician, synthetic vitamin K is not recommended during pregnancy. Too much of it can result in severe jaundice in infants as well as interference with their red blood cells.

Vitamin B group

The water-soluble B-complex vitamins, which include B_1 (thiamine), B_2 (riboflavin), B_5 (niacin), B_{12} (cobalamin), and folic acid, play an important role in tissue growth. They are found in most meats, whole wheat bread, eggs, milk, and leafy green vegetables. During pregnancy, the additional requirements for the B vitamins, except for folic acid, are quite small and are normally met by an adequate diet. The need for folic acid, however, is substantially increased because this member of the B-complex plays an important role in the growth of red blood cells. The recommended daily dose doubles from 400 milligrams to 800 milligrams in pregnancy. Since the need increases so much and since overcooking quickly destroys folic acid in many foods, the current opinion is that pregnant women should routinely receive a folic acid supplement.

Few adverse effects on either the course of pregnancy or the health of the fetus have been noted with high concentrations of the B vitamins. One report said that large amounts of vitamin B_5 (niacin) may be associated with malformations, but other researchers have not confirmed this finding.

Vitamin C

The major function of vitamin C (ascorbic acid) is in the formation of body tissues, such as skin, tendons, bone, and cartilage. It may also be involved in the absorption and use of iron and folic acid and the regulation of the cholesterol metabolism. The daily requirement is about 60 milligrams for the pregnant woman, compared to 45 milligrams for nonpregnant women. Large doses of vitamin C may adversely affect chemical processes in the fetus.

PRESCRIPTION DRUGS

A woman who is pregnant may receive a prescription for any of such an enormous number of drugs that it is not possible—in terms of space or of available knowledge—to itemize the potential consequences of all of them. What we can do here is to examine the effects of three general classes of prescription drugs that are among those frequently found in family medicine cabinets.

Amphetamines

Amphetamines are usually taken for one of two

purposes—as an antidepressant or as an appetite suppressant. More than 20 million prescriptions for amphetamines are written for American women each year, a rate four times that for men. (This figure represents only a portion of total use as amphetamines are also widely sold on the illegal drug market).

Little research has been carried out on the effects of amphetamine use during pregnancy. Animal experiments do suggest caution; when these drugs are administered during pregnancy, the offspring display a number of adverse behavioral effects, such as hyperexcitability. In humans, workers report several cases of withdrawal symptoms in infants born to amphetamine-using mothers, as well as some limited evidence linking amphetamine use to physical abnormalities.

On occasion, women have reported taking amphetamine diet pills before realizing that the weight they were putting on was attributable to pregnancy. The clear concensus of physicians is that amphetamine use should be avoided during pregnancy.

Barbiturates

Barbiturates depress the activity of the central nervous system and are used for two widely different purposes. One is in antiepileptic therapy, and in such cases they must be taken under close medical supervision. On the other hand, they are used, in a much less controlled fashion, as sleeping pills and daytime tranquilizers.

Barbiturates pass through the placenta very rapidly, and, not surprisingly since they can be highly addictive for adults, they can result in babies' being born addicted. Newborns in this situation may demonstrate withdrawal symptoms that are very marked and sometimes very long lasting. The signs of withdrawal include shaking, twitching, weakness, sleep disturbances, and convulsions, and in some cases, some of the symptoms may last several months.

Phenobarbital, perhaps the most widely used barbiturate, has been shown to pose another risk for the fetus. In addition to causing a withdrawal syndrome, its use in pregnancy has been associated with congenital anomalies, excessive fetal bleeding, and a general reduction in the responsiveness of the infant's nervous system. The baby is not able to suckle properly nor respond adequately to stimuli in the environment.

The limited available evidence indicates that barbiturates pose a considerable risk for the fetus and should be avoided in pregnancy unless they are a medical necessity.

Tranquilizers

During the past 25 years, doctors have prescribed tranquilizers in ever-increasing numbers. In fact they are so readily available that people sometimes forget they are prescription drugs and should only be used on a physician's advice.

Tranquilizers are divided into major and minor categories. The major tranquilizers are prescribed for severe mental disorders and, except in very rare circumstances, are used only under close medical supervision and when clearly dictated by the mental health of the patients. Minor tranquilizers are intended to produce calming by reducing tension and anxiety without producing sleepiness or interfering with normal mental and physical activity. Unlike barbiturates, they are presumed not to produce dependence. Over the years, however, it has become clear that use can lead to some addiction as well as to drowsiness or loss of alertness, particularly if the recommended dosage is exceeded.

Minor tranquilizers are the most commonly prescribed class of drugs. They are used regularly by an estimated six million North Americans, about two-thirds of them women. The most popular minor tranquilizers are sold under the brand names of Valium, Librium, and Miltown. The first two of these medications rank first and third respectively of all drugs prescribed in the United States and Canada.

The minor tranquilizers cross the placenta rapidly and, for unknown reasons, one hour after ingestion Valium is almost twice as concentrated in the fetal circulatory system as it is in the mother's. Because of the immaturity of the liver of the fetus and the newborn, metabolism of the drug is very slow. For example, one study showed that mothers-to-be received Valium one to three weeks before labor, the drug was still pharmacologically active in the babies for up to ten days after birth.

The infants of women who use minor tranquilizers during pregnancy may exhibit withdrawal symptoms similar to those seen among the babies born to mothers who had used other central-nervous-system depressants, such as barbiturates.

Some, but not all, researchers have found that the use of minor tranquilizers, particularly during the first trimester while the fetal organs are being formed, may increase the risk of certain malformations. Some studies have associated Valium with an increased risk of cleft palates and hare-lips, and others have linked Librium and Miltown to these anomalies as well as to cardiac abnormalities. There is also evidence that Valium interferes with the newborn's ability to regulate body temperature, causes the infant to have flaccid musculature, and may also cause a serious decrease in the breathing rate.

Although not all investigators have found these adverse associations with minor tranquilizer use during pregnancy, there is enough suggestive evidence to conclude that the mother-to-be ought not to take these drugs casually, particularly early in pregnancy, and that physicians ought to prescribe them in a circumspect fashion.

CONCLUSION

This chapter has discussed some of the most common categories of over-the-counter and prescription drugs. Obviously, it could not itemize, much less deal with, all the hundreds of thousands of products available. Even if such a compendium were attempted, the vast majority of the entries could include no information on possible effects upon pregnancy because, sadly, none is available.

Clearly, however, the facts that are available indicate that many medicines can affect the health of the unborn baby. The developing fetus receives a certain amount of the drug intended for the mother; its effects may not be the same on the fetus as on the mother, and they may last longer in the fetus than in the mother.

Thus, taking medicines during pregnancy is quite different from taking them at other times. Medication without consulting a physician ought to be avoided completely. In many cases, a nondrug remedy, such as a rest or a dietary change, may relieve the problem. If an over-the-counter drug is taken on a doctor's advice, the recommended dosage should never be exceeded.

In some situations, the health of both mother and baby warrant the use of prescription drugs. Here, the mother-to-be must rely on her doctor's advice, but various precautions are in order. First—and it is surprising how often this point is overlooked—she must make sure the doctor is aware she is pregnant. She should also tell the doctor about any drugs she is taking, on another physician's prescription or on her own initiative. Finally, she should not hesitate to discuss with her doctor the potential effects of the mediction that is being prescribed.

Expectant mothers are much more than the passive carriers of the unborn. They have an obligation to take an active, informed role in their pregnancies. Knowing the possible consequences of the medical, dietary, and social drugs that are part of a life-style is a fundamental debt owed to the unborn child.

Suggested readings

CHAPTER 1
THE FETUS AND THE NEWBORN BABY

Boston Children's Medical Center. *Pregnancy, Birth and the Newborn Baby*. New York: Dell, Delacorte Press, 1972.

Lerch, C., and V. Bliss. *Maternity Nursing*. 3rd ed. St. Louis: Mosby, 1978.
Comprehensive guides to pregnancy and childbirth with clear, approximately 20-page descriptions of the functions and structure of the placenta and some placental complications that may arise.

Brazelton, T.B. "Why Your New Baby Behaves That Way." *Redbook*, 1978, pp. 39–42.
A brief magazine article containing a description of the rationale for the Brazelton Neonatal Assessment Scale, written by the physician who originated the testing procedure.

Chamberlain, G. "The Development of the Embryo." Chap. 2 in *The Safety of the Unborn Child*. London: Penguin Hammondsworth Medical Services, 1969.
A good general description of the growth and development of different organs in the embryo and fetus.

Queenan, J.T., (ed). *A New Life, Pregnancy, Birth and Your Child's First Year*. London: Marshall Cavendish, 1979.
An overview of pregnancy, delivery, and the early growth of the child, in readable prose and with excellent drawings and photographs.

CHAPTER 2
ALCOHOL: THE ALCOHOLIC MOTHER-TO-BE

Abel, E.L. "Fetal Alcohol Syndrome: Behavioral Teratology." *Psychological Bulletin* 87 (1980): 29–50.

Randell, C.L. "Teratogenic Effects on *In Utero* Ethanol Exposure" In *Alcohol and Opiates: Neurochemical and Behavioral Mechanisms,* edited by K. Blum. New York: Academic Press, 1977. Pp. 91–107.

Reviews of many aspects of the consequences of prenatal alcohol exposure. Each article competently covers much animal work in this area.

Clarren, S.K., E.C. Alvord, Jr., M. Sumi, A.P. Steissguth, and D.W. Smith. "Brain Malformations Related to Prenatal Exposure to Ethanol." *Journal of Pediatrics* 92 (1978): 64–67.

Clarren, S.K. "Recognition of Fetal Alcohol Syndrome." *Journal of the American Medical Association* 245 (1981): 2436–39.

Two descriptions of the actual changes in the structure of the brain of children diagnosed as having the fetal alcohol syndrome. The second also gives a good account of the symptoms of the syndrome.

Jones, K.L., D.W. Smith, C.N. Ulleland, and A.P. Streissguth. "Pattern of Malformation in Offspring of Chronic Alcoholic Mothers." *Lancet* 1 (1973): 1267–71.

The original American report that described the cluster of symptoms associated with maternal alcoholism and labeled it the fetal alcohol syndrome.

Neurobehavioral Toxicology and Teratology 3 (1981), no. 2.

The issue of this journal containing papers from the Fetal Alcohol Syndrome Workshop held in Seattle, Wash. in May 1980. Included in the reports are findings from America, Canada, West Germany, and Brazil and descriptions of particular populations that are at high risk (e.g., American Indians and South Americans of low socio-economic status.) Animal research and possible biochemical causes for the syndrome are discussed, as well as several large-scale studies presently underway in Boston, Seattle, and Cleveland.

Warner, R.H., and H.L. Rosett. "The Effects of Drinking on Offspring: An Historical Survey of the American and British Literature." *Journal of Studies on Alcohol* 36 (1975): 1395–1421.
The definitive historical review of the relationship between alcohol and pregnancy.

CHAPTER 3
ALCOHOL: PREGNANCY AND SOCIAL DRINKING

Harlap, S., and P.H. Shiono. "Alcohol, Smoking and Incidence of Spontaneous Abortions in the First and Second Trimester." *Lancet* 2 (1980): 173–75.
Kline, J., P. Shrout, Z. Stein, M. Susser, and D. Warburton. "Drinking during Pregnancy and Spontaneous Abortion." *Lancet* 2 (1980): 176–80.
Back-to-back articles dealing with spontaneous abortions. The first is a report on an enormous prospective study that links increased rates of fetal loss with drinking levels of more than one drink a day. The second, a retrospective examination of the drinking habits of women who had spontaneous abortions, reports an association at consumption levels of less than one drink a day.

Kaminski, M., M. Franc, M. Lebouvier, C. duMazaubrun, and C. Rumeau-Roquette. "Moderate Alcohol Use and Pregnancy Outcome." *Neurobehavioral Toxicology and Teratology* 3 (1981): 173–81.
A description of three French studies, carried out between

1962 and 1977, that involved more than 15,000 women. The emphasis is on pregnancy outcome and fetal growth.

Mussen, P., and M.R. Rosenzweig. *Psychology: An Introduction.* 2nd ed. Lexington, Mass.: D.C. Heath, 1977.
An introductory psychology textbook with several pages devoted to a description of tests of babies, including the Bayley Scales of Infant Development.

Streissguth, A.P., D.C. Martin, J.C. Martin, and H.M. Barr. "The Seattle Longitudinal Prospective Study on Alcohol and Pregnancy." *Neurobehavioral Toxicology and Teratology* 3 (1981): 223–33.
A review of the procedures of the Seattle Pregnancy and Health Study that began in 1974, plus a summary of and references for nine completed studies in the project.

CHAPTER 4
CAFFEINE

Aranda, J.V., W. German, H. Bergsteinsson, and T. Gunn. "Efficacy of Caffeine in Treatment of Apnea in the Low-Birth-Weight Infant." *Journal of Pediatrics* 90 (1977): 467–72.
A description of the treatment with caffeine of respiratory arrest in babies.

Graham, D.M. "Caffeine — Its Identity, Dietary Sources, Intake and Biological Effects." *Nutrition Reviews* 36 (1978): 97–102.
A comprehensive, readable review of caffeine — its chemistry, commercial sources, and consumption by various age groups, and the consequences of its ingestion.

Rosenberg, L., A. Mitchell, S. Shapiro, and D. Slone. "Selected Birth Defects in Relation to Caffeine-Containing

Beverages." *The Journal of the American Medical Association* 247 (1982): 1429–32.

The report of a study that looked for and did not find an association between caffeine use during pregnancy and physical malformations.

Weathersbee, P.S., L.K. Olsen, and J.R. Lodge. "Caffeine and Pregnancy: A Retrospective Survey." *Postgraduate Medicine* 62 (1977): 64–69.

Linn, S., S. Schoenbaum, R. Monson, B. Rosner, P. Stubblefield, and K. Ryan. "No Association between Coffee Consumption and Adverse Outcomes of Pregnancy." *New England Journal of Medicine* 306 (1982): 141–45.

The Utah and Harvard studies referred to in the text. The first reports a dramatic association between heavy caffeine use and fetal loss, while the second, looking only at babies that were delivered, finds no association at more moderate levels of use.

CHAPTER 5
CIGARETTES

Abel, E.L. "Smoking during Pregnancy: A Review of Effects on Growth and Development of Offspring." *Human Biology* 52 (1980): 503–625.

A discussion of the mechanisms that may underlie prenatal growth retardation, increased risk of mortality, and behavioral abnormalities.

Fried, P.A., and H. Oxorn. *Smoking for Two: Cigarettes and Pregnancy*. New York: Free Press, 1980.

More detail, in nontechnical language, on many of the topics considered in Chapter 5. The book covers the problems associated with giving up smoking and lists alternatives to the nicotine habit. Suggested readings on a variety of topics are presented at the end of the book.

Longo, L.D. "The Biological Effects of Carbon Monoxide on the Pregnant Woman, Fetus and Newborn Infant," *American Journal of Obstetrics and Gynecology* 129 (1977): 67–103.
The definitive review of the physiological effects and clinical implications of carbon monoxide exposure in the mother-to-be and her baby.

United States Department of Health, Education, and Welfare. "Pregnancy and Infant Health." Chap. 8 in *Smoking and Health.* Washington, D.C.: U.S. Government Printing Office, 1979.
A summary of most of the recent scientific literature on birth weight and smoking, plus an extensive list of references.

CHAPTER 6
MARIJUANA

Abel, E.L. *Marijuana, the First Twelve Thousand Years.* New York: Plenum Press, 1980.
A fascinating account of the history of all aspects of marijuana, written by one of the most active researchers in the area of drug effects.

———— "Prenatal Exposure to Cannabis: A Critical Review of Effects on Growth, Development, and Behavior." *Behavioral and Neural Biology* 29 (1980): 137–56.
An up-to-date synopsis of the many animal studies of marijuana and pregnancy.

Braude, M.C., and S. Szara, eds. *Pharmacology of Marihuana.* Vol. 1 and 2. New York: Raven Press, 1976.
Nahas, G.G., and W.D.M. Paton, eds. *Marihuana: Biological Effects, Analysis, Metabolism, Cellular Responses, Reproduction and Brain.* Oxford: Pergamon Press, 1979.

Peterson, R.C., ed. *Marijuana Research Findings: 1980.* NIDA Research Monograph 31. Washington: U.S. Government Printing Office
A large number of reports by researchers around the world, representing current knowledge of the effects of marijuana on animal and human systems.

Fried, P.A., B. Watkinson, A. Grant, and R.M. Knights. "Changing Patterns of Soft Drug Use prior to and during Pregnancy: A Prospective Study." *Drug and Alcohol Dependence* 6 (1980): 323–43.

Fried, P.A. "Marihuana Use by Pregnant Women: Neurobehavioral Effects in Neonates." *Drug and Alcohol Dependence* 6 (1980): 415–24.

—— "Marihuana Use by Pregnant Women and Effects on Offspring: An Update." *Neurobehavioral Toxicology and Teratology* (1982):
Three articles describing the ongoing Ottawa study referred to Chapter 6. They give details on the soft drugs used by the women and some of the results found in the newborn and young babies.

CHAPTER 7
NONPRESCRIPTION AND PRESCRIPTION MEDICINES

Collins, E. "Maternal and Fetal Effects of Acetaminophen and Salicylates in Pregnancy." *Obstetrics & Gynecology* 58 (1981 supplement): 57–62.
A recent review of the effects of painkillers on both the mother and the fetus. Some animal work is described.

Finnegan, L.P., and K.O. Fehr. "The Effects of Opiates, Sedative-Hypnotics, Amphetamines, Cannabis, and Other Psychoactive Drugs on the Fetus and Newborn." In *Alcohol and Drug Problems in Women,* Vol. 5, edited by O.J. Kalant. New York; Plenum Press, 1980. Pp. 653–723.
A lengthy chapter provides a description of drug use

during pregnancy by women around the world. It gives in considerable detail the effects of the various drugs named in the title and presents an interesting discussion of the clinical management of both mother and child.

Moghissi, K.S. "Risks and Benefits of Nutritional Supplements during Pregnancy." *Obstetrics & Gynecology* 58 (1981 supplement) 68–78.
A review emphasizing the role of minerals and vitamins in pregnancy. It includes discussion of the dietary sources of these nutrients, the requirements during pregnancy, and whether there is a need for supplements.

Glossary

ABORTION
See Spontaneous Abortion.

ABRUPTIO PLACENTA
The premature detachment of the placenta from the wall of the uterus, resulting in the interruption of the oxygen supply to the fetus. If the separation is large, the fetus cannot survive, but if only a small area has detached, rapid delivery, usually by cesarean section, can produce a live baby.

ABSTINENCE SYNDROME
See Withdrawal

ADDICTION
Compulsive use of a habit-forming drug.

ALCOHOLISM
Intermittent or continuous use of alcohol associated with dependency, psychological or physical. The behavioral disorders that arise from the excessive consumption are of such degree that they interfere with the drinker's mental and physical health.

AMNIOTIC FLUID
A fluid, derived primarily from a filtrate of the mother's blood, in which the embryo floats. At term, the volume is 16 to 32 ounces.

ANALGESICS
Drugs or other agents that relieve pain without causing loss of consciousness.

ANEMIA
A reduction in the red blood cells below the normal level.

APGAR TEST
A numerical assessment of the condition of the baby at birth, made at one minute and again at five minutes of age. The baby is assigned points for each of five items: (1) heart rate; (2) respiratory effort; (3) muscle tone; (4) reflex responsiveness; and (5) color.

AROUSAL
A state of responsiveness to sensory stimulation.

BLOOD-BRAIN BARRIER
A mechanism that prevents potentially harmful chemicals in the blood from reaching the brain.

BINGE DRINKING
Consumption of a large number of drinks over a short period of time.

CESAREAN SECTION
An operation in which the baby is lifted directly from the uterus through an incision made in the abdomen and uterus.

CLEFT PALATE
A fissure or an opening of the roof of the mouth sometimes present at birth. Often combined with harelip.

CIRRHOSIS
Inflamation of an organ, particularly the liver.

CONGENITAL MALFORMATION
A malformation that is present at and exists from the time of birth.

DISTILLATION
The conversion, by heating, of a liquid into vapors, which are then cooled and reconverted to liquid by condensation. The substances that evaporate more

quickly are collected and the impurities remain in the residue.

DOSE RESPONSE
The relationship between the dosage or amount of a particular drug and the action or change it causes. The effect usually becomes more pronounced as the quantity of the drug increases.

EMBRYO
A developing baby; in humans, the first eight weeks of intrauterine existence. The organs are formed during this period.

ENZYMES
Chemicals, existing in cells, that speed up such reactions as the metabolism of alcohol. Enzymes remain unchanged during their participation in chemical reactions.

FALLOPIAN TUBES
Tubes, one on each side of the pelvic cavity, that are attached at one end to the uterus; the other, unattached ends lie close to the ovaries. One tube conducts the egg from the ovary to the interior of the uterus.

FETUS
A developing baby; for humans, the last 32 weeks of intrauterine life. During this period, the organ structures laid down in the earlier (embryonic) stage are developed, and the baby prepares to change from the fluid environment of the uterus to life in air, separate from its mother.

FRATERNAL TWINS
Two offspring produced in one pregnancy but developed from two separate ova fertilized at more or less the same time by separate sperm. The genetic makeups are no more similar than those of siblings born years apart.

GENES
Small entities, lying on chromosomes, that are the

biologic units of heredity. They provide the basic hereditary information and controls and account for inherited individual differences. Genes are composed of the biochemical substance deoxyribonucleic acid (DNA).

GESTATION

The period of development of the baby from the time of fertilization until birth. In humans, the normal gestation period is approximately 266 days from successful coitus or about 280 days (40 weeks) from the first day of the last normal menstrual period.

HABITUATION

Becoming used to a new stimulus so that it no longer seems notable or upsetting.

HARELIP

Also called a cleft lip. A notch in the upper lip as a result of incomplete closure during embryonic development. Frequently present in conjunction with a cleft palate.

HASHISH

Resin from the marijuana plant with a high (5 to 10 percent) THC content.

HEMP

The term used for the marijuana plant when it is grown primarily for its tough fiber, which is used to make rope, sailcloth, and clothing.

HEMOGLOBIN

An iron-containing protein in red blood cells that is capable of carrying oxygen to the tissues.

HEMORRHAGE

The escape of blood from blood vessels.

HORMONES

Substances that act as chemical messengers in the blood, stimulating the body's cells to perform their functions.

HYPERACTIVITY
A disorder of childhood, usually disappearing during adolescence, marked by overactivity, distractibility, restlessness, and low tolerance for frustration.

IDENTICAL TWIN
Two offspring produced in one pregnancy and developed from one fertilized ovum. The genetic makeup is identical for the two individuals.

INVOLUNTARY SMOKING
The inhalation by a nonsmoker of the products contained in the atmosphere of a smoke-filled environment.

JAUNDICE
A yellowish tinge of the skin resulting from the accumulation of the pigment biliruben. Before birth, biliruben is secreted across the placenta and excreted by the mother's liver. After birth, the baby's own liver must excrete it but usually does not do so for several days.

JOINT
A marijuana cigarette.

LIPOPROTEIN
Any of a group of organic compounds consisting of fats and proteins. They are insoluble in water and soluble in fat solvents and alcohol.

METABOLIZATION
The chemical processes in living cells by which substances are altered so that they can be used by the body or broken down as waste products.

MORO REFLEX
A reflex set off in the newborn by a sudden motion. It is a startle response consisting of the throwing out of the arms and spreading of the hands; this extension is followed by the closing of the hands and a bringing together of the arms with the effect of clasping anyone or anything within reach.

MOTOR SYSTEM
The structures in the body that control and produce movements. They include structures in the brain, nerves, and muscles.

NEONATE
The term used to describe an infant from birth to about four weeks of age.

NEURON
A nerve cell; a form of cell with long branching processes specialized to generate and conduct electrochemical signals. It is the basic unit of the nervous system in all animals.

OVUM (plural: OVA)
An egg. The female reproductive cell, which, after fertilization, is capable of developing into a new member of the same species.

PASSIVE SMOKING
See Involuntary Smoking.

PLACENTA
Tissue joining the mother and the offspring during pregnancy. On the mother's side, it is in contact with the wall of the uterus; via the placenta, oxygen, nutrients and waste products are exchanged. After delivery, the placenta (frequently called the afterbirth) is expelled.

POLYDRUG USER
An individual who uses many drugs.

PREMATURE BABY
A baby born after a pregnancy of less than 37 weeks.

PROBABILITY
A measure of predictability with respect to some future event. Probability is the long-run expectation of the relative frequency with which a given event will occur.

PROOF
Alcoholic strength of a liquid. It is designated as twice the percentage of alcohol by volume. Thus, a whisky labeled 80 proof contains 40 percent alcohol.

PROSPECTIVE RESEARCH
Research that gathers information as it becomes available. The obtained facts are used to determine whether any of the information is predictive of particular complications or behavior.

REFLEX
An automatic, stereotyped response that arises as a direct result of a stimulus.

RESPIRATORY DISTRESS
A condition affecting premature babies in which the lungs collapse with each expiration, making breathing more difficult and less efficient.

RETROSPECTIVE RESEARCH
Research that looks backward to what has been experienced in the past. Frequently, it is undertaken once a behavior or compliction has been identified and researchers are trying to establish its cause.

RISK FACTOR
The likelihood or probability, based on available studies and/or statistics, that a particular stimulus (e.g., alcohol) will cause a particular event (e.g., mental retardation).

ROOTING REFLEX
The baby's turning of the head and movements of lips in response to gentle stroking of the cheek.

SOCIAL DRINKING
Drinking alcoholic beverages in an amount that society does not consider excessive. There is no universal definition as norms vary from society to society. In North America, it generally means an average consumption of

no more than two drinks per day and rarely more than one or two drinks per drinking occasion.

SPONTANEOUS ABORTION
The natural expulsion from the uterus of either the embryo or fetus before the offspring is mature enough to survive.

STILLBIRTH
The delivery of a dead baby.

TEMPERANCE
Moderation in drinking alcoholic beverages. However, since the 19th century, some "temperance" groups have preached complete abstinence from alcohol.

TERATOGEN
A substance that has the capacity of affecting normal intrauterine development resulting in physical malformations and/or behavioral anomalies.

TERM
The average length of human pregnancy: 280 days from the first day of the last menstrual period. A full-term pregnancy is one that ends in delivery after 259 to 293 days (37 to 42 weeks).

THC (1-delta-9-tetrahydrocannabinol)
The active ingredient in marijuana that, in high enough doses, causes hallucination.

TONE
The normal degree of vigor and tension in a muscle. It is often measured by the muscle's resistance to somebody else's trying to stretch it.

TRIMESTER
One of three three-month periods into a which a pregnancy is divided.

ULTRASOUND
An apparently safe technique that has replaced the X-rays as a way of looking at the development of the pregnancy in the uterus. It uses sound waves of such a high frequency that they cannot be heard.

UMBILICAL CORD
The link between the placenta and the abdominal region of the fetus. It contains two arteries (carrying blood and waste products from the baby to the placenta) and one vein (transporting oxygen- and nutrient-carrying blood from the placenta to the baby).

UTERUS
The hollow organ, suspended in the cavity of the pelvis, in which the fetus grows.

VILLI (PLACENTAL)
Fingerlike projections from the fetal side of the placenta that are bathed in the mother's blood in the uterus. The transfer between mother and baby takes place through the walls of the villi.

WITHDRAWAL SYMPTOMS
A physiological and behavioral reaction, sometimes severe, that takes place when drug use is abruptly terminated.

WOMB
See Uterus.

Index